Collins

Calorie Counter

SCOTLAND*on*SUNDAY

This book has been compiled with the assistance of hundreds of brand-name manufacturers and from the major supermarkets. Values for unbranded foods have been obtained from *The Composition of Foods* (5th edition, 1991 and 6th summary edition, 2002) and *Vegetables, Herbs and Spices* (supplement, 1991), and have been reproduced by permission of Controller of Her Majesty's Stationery Office. The publishers are grateful to all manufacturers who gave information on their products. If you cannot find a particular food here, you can obtain much fuller listings of nutrient counts in branded foods from the *Collins Gem Calorie Counter*.

HarperCollins Publishers
Westerhill Road, Bishopbriggs
Glasgow G64 2QT

The Collins website is www.collins.co.uk

This edition produced especially for Scotland on Sunday

© HarperCollins Publishers 2006

ISBN 0 00 776198-8

Printed and bound in Great Britain by
Bookmarque Ltd, Croydon, Surrey

CONTENTS

HOW TO USE THIS BOOK

The foods in this book are grouped into categories
– Bakery, Biscuits, Condiments & Sauces, etc. – and
listed in alphabetical order in the left-hand column
of each page, together with portion sizes and
cooking methods, where applicable. The portion
sizes given are 'average' ones that you might eat
in a single serving, such as one medium apple, or
100g of chicken breast. We have also used cup
measurements where they are helpful, because
it's easier to visualise a cup of salad than to weigh
out a specific weight of lettuce leaves, especially
if you are eating in a restaurant. Note: think of a
teacup-full rather than a huge mug!

The first column gives the Calorie count of the
food in kilocalories (abbreviated to kcal). Note
that 1 Calorie (with a capital C) is the same as
1 kilocalorie. The remaining columns give the
carbohydrate, fibre, protein and fat content of
the portion in grams. Note that values are given
for cooked products rather than raw. Pasta, rice
and pulses swell up to approximately three times
their weight when cooked, but food packaging
often gives the values for their dry weight. Read
the weights on the packaging of any ready-
prepared food as portion sizes will vary from
product to product.

Here's a quick formula for calculating roughly how many Calories you can consume in a day without gaining weight:

- If you are a woman with a largely sedentary lifestyle (desk job, car, little time to exercise), multiply your weight in kilos by 26 to get the number of calories you should eat a day to maintain your current weight.
- If you are a sedentary man, multiply your weight in kg by 31.
- If you are an active woman (getting 60 minutes of moderate-intensity exercise a day plus three sessions of aerobic exercise a week), multiply your weight in kg by 33.
- If you are an active man, multiply your weight in kg by 37.
- If you are a very active woman (getting 60 minutes of moderate-intensity exercise a day plus five to seven sessions of aerobic exercise a week), multiply your weight in kg by 39.
- If you are a very active man, multiply your weight in kg by 44.

It has been calculated that a kilogram of weight is equivalent to 7,700 Calories, so for every kilo a dieter wants to lose, 7,700 Calories must be cut from the diet or burned through exercise (or preferably both). Sensible weight loss to aim at is around 0.5 kg a week, and to achieve this you would have to consume 3,350 calories fewer a week – or 478 fewer a day.

CONVERSION CHART

Metric to imperial

100 grams (g) = 3.53 ounces (oz)
1 kilogram (kg) = 2.2 pounds (lb)
100 millilitres (ml) = 3.38 fluid ounces (fl oz)
1 litre = 1.76 pints

Imperial to metric

1 ounce (oz) = 28.35 grams (g)
1 pound (lb) = 453.6 grams (g)
1 stone (st) = 6.35 kilograms (kg)
1 fluid ounce (fl oz) = 29.57 millilitres (ml)
1 pint = 0.568 litres (l)

Abbreviations used in the listings

g	gram
kcal	kilocalorie
ml	millilitre
Tr	trace
n/a	figures not available
—	none
cal	calories
carb	carbohydrate
pro	protein

Bakery	Cal (kcal)	Carb (g)	Fibre (g)	Pro (g)	Fat (g)
Bread					
Brown, 1 slice	62	12.6	1.5	2.4	0.6
Brown, toasted, 1 slice	82	17.0	2.1	3.1	0.6
Chapattis:					
made with fat, each (50g)	164	24.2	n/a	4.1	6.4
made without fat, each (50g)	101	21.9	n/a	3.7	0.5
Ciabatta, 1 slice	81	15.5	1.0	3.0	1.2
Currant loaf, 1 slice	87	15.3	n/a	2.3	2.3
French stick, 1 slice (2cm thick)	88	18.7	1.1	3.0	0.6
Garlic bread, pre-packed, frozen, 1 slice	110	13.6	–	2.4	5.5
Granary, 1 slice	71	14.1	1.6	2.9	0.7
High-bran, 1 slice	64	10.2	2.4	4.0	0.8
Malt, 1 slice	88	19.4	1.0	2.3	0.7
Naan, plain, half	177	31.2	1.8	4.9	4.5
Oatmeal, 1 slice	70	12.4	1.1	2.4	1.2
Pitta bread, white, medium:	128	27.7	1.2	4.6	0.7
white with sesame	131	24	1.5	4.8	1.8
wholewheat	114	20.5	3.1	5.4	1.2
Pitta bread, 2 mini (10g each)	52	11.4	0.7	1.7	0.3
Pumpernickel, 1 slice	68	14.1	1.7	2.3	0.5
Rye, 1 slice	66	13.8	n/a	2.5	0.5
Sourdough, 1 slice	78	14.7	0.9	2.5	0.9
Stoneground wholemeal, 1 slice	65	11.8	2.2	2.9	0.7

Bakery	Cal (kcal)	Carb (g)	Fibre (g)	Pro (g)	Fat (g)
Wheatgerm, 1 slice	66	11.9	1.7	3.4	0.9
White, 1 slice	66	13.9	0.8	2.4	0.5
White, fried in oil/lard, 1 slice	149	14.0	0.8	2.4	9.7
White, toasted, 1 slice	81	17.0	0.9	2.9	0.6
Wholemeal, 1 slice	66	12.7	2.1	2.8	0.8
Rolls					
Bagels, each (70g):	192	37.2	1.5	7.8	1.0
onion bagels	192	37.7	1.5	7.8	1.1
sesame bagels	190	36.9	1.5	7.9	1.3
cinnamon & raisin	197	39.2	1.5	7.4	1.3
Baps, white, each (60g)	141	26.2	1.6	5.9	2.6
Brown, crusty, each (60g)	153	30.2	n/a	6.2	1.7
Brown, soft, each (60g)	142	26.9	2.6	5.9	1.9
Hamburger bun, each (60g)	158	29.2	n/a	5.4	3
White, crusty, each (60g)	157	32.9	1.7	5.5	1.3
White, soft, each (60g)	153	30.9	1.6	5.6	1.6
Wholemeal, each (60g)	147	27.7	3.3	6.3	2.0
Taco shells, each (30g)	152	18.4	n/a	2.1	7.8
Tortillas, each (30g):					
corn	103	18.1	n/a	3.0	2.1
flour	97	15.7	n/a	2.7	2.7

TIP: Brown bread is often made with normal white flour, but coloured with caramel or molasses. Opt for wholemeal instead.

Bakery	Cal (kcal)	Carb (g)	Fibre (g)	Pro (g)	Fat (g)
Tea Breads, Buns, Pastries					
Brioche, each (60g)	208	32.9	1.3	4.8	6.3
Chelsea bun, each (70g)	257	39.0	n/a	5.5	9.9
Croissant, each (70g)	261	30.3	2.2	5.8	13.8
Crumpet, each (50g)	91	15.9	1.5	3.0	0.4
Currant bun, each (70g)	196	36.8	2.0	5.6	3.9
Danish pastry, each (70g)	240	35.9	–	4.1	9.9
Doughnut, each (70g):					
jam	235	34.1	n/a	4.0	10.1
ring	282	33.1	–	4.3	15.7
Eccles cake, each (60g)	232	33.8	n/a	2.4	10.7
Fruit loaf, slice (70g)	217	44.9	n/a	4.9	3.4
Hot cross bun, each (70g)	218	40.9	n/a	5.2	4.9
Muffin, each (70g):					
English	160	29.5	2.3	7.1	1.5
blueberry	300	34.9	0.8	3	0.8
Potato scone, each (60g)	124	25.2	2.6	2.8	1.3
Raisin and cinnamon					
loaf, slice (70g)	182	35	2.2	4.9	2.9
Scone, each (60g):					
fruit	207	30.7	1.7	4.8	7.2

TIP: Slice bread then freeze it. You're much less likely to snack on frozen bread, but individual slices can be toasted straight from the freezer when you really need them.

Bakery	Cal (kcal)	Carb (g)	Fibre (g)	Pro (g)	Fat (g)
Scones *contd:*					
plain	218	32.2	n/a	4.3	8.9
wholemeal	197	25.9	n/a	5.3	8.8
Scotch pancake, each (60g)	158	29.8	0.7	4.0	2.7
Cakes and Cream Cakes					
Almond slice (50g bar)	212	20.6	0.8	6.5	12.9
Apple Danish (50g bar)	165	20.7	1.1	3.3	7.8
Bakewell slice (50g)	150	19.4	0.4	1.5	7.4
Banana cake, slice (75g)	260	41.9	0.5	2.4	6
Battenburg, slice (75g)	323	52.7	1.0	5.2	10.1
Brownies, chocolate, each (75g)	365	40.6	1.6	3.8	20.7
Caramel shortcake, piece (50g)	248	27.6	0.5	2	14.5
Carrot cake, slice (75g)	300	44.9	0.9	2.4	12.3
Chocolate cake, slice (75g)	268	42.3	1	4.3	10.5
Chocolate mini roll, each (50g)	222	27.4	0.7	2.2	11.1
Chocolate sandwich sponge, slice (50g)	192	24.0	0.9	2.0	9.8
Date and walnut loaf, slice (75g)	264	30.8	0.8	4.4	13.7

TIP: If you crave cake, choose a slice of fruit loaf. Many are fat-free – but don't spread it with butter.

Bakery	Cal (kcal)	Carb (g)	Fibre (g)	Pro (g)	Fat (g)
Chocolate éclair, each (75g)	297	19.6	n/a	4.2	23.0
Fancy cake, iced, each (50g)	178	34.5	–	1.9	4.6
Flapjack, oat, each (75g)	370	46.8	n/a	3.6	20.3
Fruit cake, slice (75g):					
plain	278	43.4	–	3.8	11.1
rich	257	44.9	n/a	2.9	8.5
rich, iced	263	49.4	–	2.7	7.4
wholemeal	274	39.3	n/a	4.5	12.1
Ginger cake, slice (75g)	295	46.4	0.9	2.6	11.0
Greek pastries (sweet), each (50g)	161	20	–	2.4	8.5
Lemon cake, slice (75g)	289	41.6	0.8	3.4	13.5
Marble cake, slice (75g)	278	41.6	0.9	3.9	10.5
Madeira cake, slice (75g)	283	43.8	–	4.1	11.3
Mince pie, each (50g)	198	30	0.8	1.9	7.8
Sponge cake, slice (50g):					
plain	234	26.3	n/a	3.2	13.6
fat-free	151	26.5	n/a	5	3.5
jam-filled	151	32.1	n/a	2.1	2.5
with butter icing	245	26.2	0.3	2.3	15.5
Swiss roll, original, slice (50g)	146	30.3	0.6	2.6	1.6
Trifle sponge, each (50g)	162	33.6	0.5	2.6	2.0

TIP: Be careful what you eat with your bread. Think about the fat level – and type of fat – of anything you spread on it.

Beans, Pulses & Cereals	Cal (kcal)	Carb (g)	Fibre (g)	Pro (g)	Fat (g)
Beans and Pulses					
Aduki beans, 115g	141	25.9	n/a	10.7	0.2
Baked beans, small can (200g):					
in tomato sauce	168	30.6	n/a	10.4	1.2
tomato sauce, no added sugar	132	22.6	7.4	9.4	0.4
Baked beans with pork sausages, small can (200g)	194	22.0	6.0	11.2	6.8
Baked beans with vegetable sausages, small can (200g)	210	24.4	5.8	12.0	7.2
Blackeyed beans, 115g	133	22.9	n/a	10.1	0.8
Borlotti beans, half can (100g)	121	20.5	5.5	8.7	0.5
Broad beans, small can (200g)	164	22	10	16	1.4
Butter beans:					
small can (200g)	166	27.8	9.6	12.0	0.8
dried, boiled (115g)	118	21.2	6	8.2	0.7
Cannellini beans, *small can* (200g)	174	28	12	14	0.6
Chick peas:					
small can (200g)	230	32.2	n/a	14.4	5.8
dried, boiled (115g)	139	20.9	n/a	9.7	2.4

TIP: A fresh lentil salad, with a little raw red onion and fresh herbs mixed with the cooked lentils, is delicious. Mix an oil and vinegar dressing at least 30 minutes before serving so the flavours can develop.

Beans, Pulses & Cereals	Cal (kcal)	Carb (g)	Fibre (g)	Pro (g)	Fat (g)
Chilli beans, small can (200g)	160	28	7.4	9.6	1
Flageolet beans, half can (100g)	132	22.4	2.4	9.0	0.7
Haricot beans, 115g					
dried, boiled	109	19.8	7	7.6	0.6
Hummus, 2 tbsp	53	3.3	n/a	2.2	3.6
Lentils, 115g:					
green/brown, boiled	121	19.4	n/a	10.1	0.8
red, split, boiled	115	20.1	n/a	8.7	0.5
Marrow fat peas:					
small can (200g)	168	28	9.6	12	0.8
quick-soak, 115g	334	48.2	16.1	29.1	2.8
Mung beans, 115g					
boiled	105	17.6	n/a	8.7	0.5
Pinto beans:					
boiled, 115g	158	27.5	–	10.2	0.8
refried, 2 tbsp	32	4.6	–	1.9	0.3
Red kidney beans:					
small can (200g)	182	27	12.8	16.2	1.0
boiled, 115g	118	20	n/a	9.7	0.6
Soya beans, 115g					
dried, boiled	162	5.9	n/a	16.1	8.4

TIP: Try using soaked and cooked dried beans, or tinned ones, to replace some of the meat in family favourites like shepherd's pie, stews, moussaka or lasagne.

Beans, Pulses & Cereals	Cal (kcal)	Carb (g)	Fibre (g)	Pro (g)	Fat (g)
Split peas, 115g, *boiled*	145	26.1	3.1	9.5	1
Tofu (soya bean curd), 2 tbsp:					
steamed	94	0.9	–	10.4	5.4
fried	337	2.6	–	30.3	22.9
Cereals					
Barley, pearl, 100g	360	83.6	7.3	7.9	1.7
Bran, 100g:					
wheat, dry	206	26.8	n/a	14.1	5.5
Bulgur wheat, dry, 100g	357	74	3.1	12	1.4
Couscous, dry, 100g	355	72.5	2	13.5	1.9
Cracked wheat, 100g	357	74	3.1	12	1.4
Polenta, ready-made, 100g	72	15.7	n/a	1.6	0.3
Wheatgerm, 100g	357	44.7	n/a	26.7	9.2

Fresh beans & peas:
see Vegetables
For more soya products:
see Vegetarian

TIP: You can keep dried beans for years but they get drier and harder as they get older, becoming resistant to soaking and cooking. It's best to buy small quantities at a time, and don't buy any packs that look dusty. Keep beans in airtight containers.

Biscuits & Crackers	Cal (kcal)	Carb (g)	Fibre (g)	Pro (g)	Fat (g)
Sweet Biscuits					
Bourbon creams, each	47	7	n/a	n/a	1.9
Caramel wafers, each	45	6.7	n/a	0.5	2
Chocolate chip cookies, each	43	5.7	n/a	0.6	2
Chocolate cream wafers, each	26	3.2	n/a	0.3	1.4
Chocolate fingers, each:					
milk & plain chocolate	52	6.3	n/a	0.7	2.7
white chocolate	53	6.1	n/a	0.6	3
Shortcake cream sandwich					
fruit	75	9.2	0.3	0.9	3.8
milk chocolate	77	9.4	0.3	0.9	3.9
mint	78	9.4	0.3	0.8	4
orange	78	9.3	0.3	0.8	4.1
Custard creams, each	51	6.9	0.2	0.6	2.3
Digestive biscuits, each:					
uncoated	58	8.6	–	0.8	2.5
chocolate (milk & plain)	74	10	–	1	3.6
Fig rolls each	36	6.8	0.5	0.4	0.8
Garibaldi (plain), each	40	7.1	0.3	0.5	1.0
Gingernuts, each	44	8	–	0.6	1.3
Gipsy creams, each	77	9.9	0.4	0.7	3.8
Jaffa cakes, each	37	7.0	0.2	0.5	0.8
Lemon puff, each	52	6.2	0.2	0.7	2.7
Nice biscuits, each	49	6.9	0.2	0.7	2.1
Oat & raisin biscuits, each	47	6.3	0.4	0.8	2.1

Biscuits & Crackers	Cal (kcal)	Carb (g)	Fibre (g)	Pro (g)	Fat (g)
Rich tea biscuits, each	46	7.2	0.3	0.7	1.6
Shortbread fingers, each	100	12.8	0.4	1.2	5.2
Shortcake biscuits, each	49	6.5	n/a	0.6	2.3
Stem ginger cookies, diet, each	40	6.5	0.1	0.5	1.3
Viennese whirls, each	21	2.3	0.1	0.2	1.3
Wafer biscuits, cream-filled, each	37	4.6	–	0.3	2.1
Crackers and Crispbreads					
Bran crackers, 4	91	12.6	0.6	1.9	3.6
Cheese crackers , 4	81	8.3	0.4	1.5	4.7
Cornish wafers, each	53	5.4	0.2	0.8	3.1
Cream crackers, each	36	5.7	0.3	0.8	1.1
Oatcakes, each:					
fine	46	6.3	0.9	1	2.2
organic	42	7.1	0.9	0.9	1.6
rough	43	6.4	0.8	1.2	1.8
traditional	43	5.8	0.8	1.1	1.7
Rye crispbread, each:					
dark rye	31	6.5	1.8	0.9	0.1
multigrain	33	5.7	1.7	1.1	0.6
original	33	6.7	1.7	1.1	0.1
Water biscuits, 3:					
regular (table)	41	7.5	0.4	1	0.8
Wholemeal crackers, 4	62	10.8	0.7	1.5	1.7

Breakfast Cereals & Bars	Cal (kcal)	Carb (g)	Fibre (g)	Pro (g)	Fat (g)
Breakfast Cereals					
Bran flakes, 30g	97	19.8	4.5	3	0.6
Cheerios, 40g:	148	30.1	2.6	3.2	1.6
honey-nut	150	31.3	2.1	2.8	1.5
Cornflakes, 30g:	112	23.4	0.9	2.1	0.3
Crunchy nut	18	24.9	0.8	11.8	1.2
Sugar coated	111	26.1	0.6	1.4	0.2
Chocolate sugar coated	118	24.0	1.1	1.5	1.8
Fruit 'n' Fibre, 30g	107	20.4	2.7	2.4	1.8
Grape Nuts, 40g	138	29	3.4	4.2	0.8
High Fibre Bran, 40g	112	18.4	10.8	5.6	1.8
Low fat flakes, 30g:	112	22.5	0.8	4.8	0.3
with red berries	111	22.8	0.9	4.2	0.3
Malted Wheats, 30g	108	21.9	2.8	3.2	0.8
Multi-grain cereal, 30g	113	24	1.5	2.4	0.8
Oat Bran Flakes, 30g	99	20.1	0.6	3	0.6
Oat Krunchies, 30g	108	18.9	3.3	3.2	2.1
Puffed Rice, 30g:	114	26.1	0.3	1.8	0.3
chocolate	115	25.2	0.6	1.5	0.9
sugar coated	115	27	0.3	1.4	0.2
Puffed Wheat, 30g	98	18.7	1.7	4.6	0.4

TIP: Put porridge on to cook while you get on with your morning tasks, but remember to stir it occasionally. You will learn to judge how much you can do – perhaps washing and dressing – before it is ready.

Breakfast Cereals & Bars	Cal (kcal)	Carb (g)	Fibre (g)	Pro (g)	Fat (g)
Shredded wheat bisks, 30g:	102	20.3	3.5	3.5	0.8
bitesize	105	21.0	3.6	3.5	0.8
sugar coated	105	21.6	2.7	3	0.6
fruit-filled	106	20.6	2.7	2.5	1.5
honey nut	113	20.6	2.8	3.4	2
Sultana Bran, 30g	95	20.1	0.4	2.4	0.6
Wheat bisks, 30g	101	20.4	3.0	3.5	0.6
Hot Cereals					
Instant Porridge					
baked apple	374	71	5.5	8	6
berry burst	374	71	5.5	8	6
golden syrup	372	71	6	7.5	6
Oatbran, 100g	345	49.7	15.2	14.8	9.7
Oatmeal, medium or fine, 100g	359	60.4	8.5	11	8.1
Oats, 100g:					
instant	359	60.4	8.5	11	8.1
jumbo	359	60.4	8.5	11	8.1
organic	363	61.5	8.0	12.5	7.4
rolled	368	62	7	11	8

TIP: A couple of apples and a handful of nuts are a better choice than a cereal bar. Most cereal bars on the market are sugar-coated and often have extra sweeteners on top. Muesli bars with dried fruits and seeds may look healthy but can also be loaded with sugar.

Breakfast Cereals & Bars	Cal (kcal)	Carb (g)	Fibre (g)	Pro (g)	Fat (g)
Porridge (cooked), 100g:					
made with water	46	8.1	n/a	1.4	1.1
made with whole milk	113	12.6	n/a	4.8	5.1
Muesli					
Crunchy Oat Cereal, 50g:					
maple & pecan	224	30.0	3.3	5	9.4
raisin & almond	211	33	2.8	3.5	7.2
sultana & apple	189	29.6	6.2	3.8	6.1
Muesli, 50g:	182	33	3.8	5	3.4
apricot	142	29.5	2.8	3.9	1.8
deluxe	172	28.1	5.8	5.4	5
high fibre	158	35.4	3	5.2	3
natural	173	31.5	4.3	4.8	3.1
organic	177	29.8	4.5	4.5	4.4
swiss-style	182	36.1	n/a	4.9	3
swiss-style, organic	180	31.5	3.7	4.9	3.8
with no added sugar	183	33.6	n/a	5.3	3.9

TIP: Make your own muesli. Mix 450g porridge oats with 50g oat bran, 2 tablespoons each of sunflower seeds, pumpkin seeds and chopped nuts, plus a tablespoon of linseed. For toasted muesli, put this mixture in an ovenproof dish and bake at 200°C/gas mark 6 for about 15 minutes until it looks golden; stir once during this time. Once it has cooled add 50g chopped dried apricots. Mix well and store in an airtight jar.

Breakfast Cereals & Bars	Cal (kcal)	Carb (g)	Fibre (g)	Pro (g)	Fat (g)
Cereal Bars					
Apple & blackberry, 30g	117	20.8	1.5	1.6	3.1
Banana, 30g	152	27.6	2	2.3	2
Cornflakes & milk bar, 30g	132	19.8	0.6	2.7	4.8
Fruit & Nut Break, 30g	170	23.7	2	3.0	7.0
Fruit and oats crisp, 30g:					
Apricot	122	21.3	2.1	1.7	3.3
Raisin & Hazelnut	142	20.4	1.3	2.1	5.8
Low fat flakes & milk bar, 30g	135	20.7	0.4	2.1	4.8
Muesli bar, 30g	178	30.6	2	2.7	5
Multi-grain bar, 30g:					
Apple	106	19.8	1.1	1.2	2.7
Cappuccino	111	19.8	0.7	1.4	3
Cherry	104	20.1	1.2	1.2	2.4
Chocolate	110	19.8	1.2	1.4	3.0
Orange	105	19.5	1.2	1.2	2.7
Strawberry	107	20.1	1.1	1.2	2.7
Oat and wheat bar, 30g:	117	22.5	0.6	2.1	2.1
Chocolate chip	147	17.7	0.5	2.1	7.2
Roasted nut	151	16.4	0.4	2.7	8

TIP: Most breakfast cereals have a lot of added sugar, even some of the 'healthy' or 'vitamin-enriched' ones. Go for those based on bran or oats, but still check labels carefully. Top them with skimmed milk, or low-fat, unsweetened soya milk with added calcium.

Condiments & Sauces	Cal (kcal)	Carb (g)	Fibre (g)	Pro (g)	Fat (g)
Table Sauces					
Apple sauce, 1 tbsp	16	4	0.2	–	Tr
Barbecue sauce, 1 tbsp	18	4.1	0.1	0.1	–
Beetroot in redcurrant jelly					
1 tbsp	25	6.1	n/a	0.1	Tr
Brown fruity sauce, 1 tbsp	17	3.6	0.2	0.1	–
Brown sauce, 1 tbsp	15	3.4	n/a	0.2	–
Burger sauce, 1 tbsp	36	1.8	Tr	0.2	3.1
Chilli sauce, 1 tsp	7	1.7	–	0.1	Tr
Cranberry jelly, 1 tbsp	40	10	–	Tr	Tr
Cranberry sauce, 1 tbsp	27	6.8	n/a	–	–
Garlic sauce, 1 tsp	17	0.9	n/a	0.1	1.5
Ginger sauce, 1 tsp	6	1.4	–	–	–
Horseradish, creamed, 2 tsp	18	2	0.2	0.2	1
Horseradish relish, 2 tsp	11	1	0.3	0.2	0.6
Horseradish sauce, 2 tsp	15	1.8	n/a	0.2	0.8
Mint jelly, 1 tbsp	40	10	n/a	Tr	–
Mint sauce, 1 tbsp	9	1.9	n/a	0.2	–
Mushroom ketchup, 1 tbsp	4	0.8	Tr	0.1	–
Redcurrant jelly, 1 tbsp	39	9.8	n/a	–	–
Soy sauce, 2 tsp	4	0.8	n/a	0.3	Tr

TIP: Make your own apple sauce by blending some unsweetened stewed apples until they are still slightly rough in texture. The better the quality of the apples you use, the better your sauce will be.

Condiments & Sauces	Cal (kcal)	Carb (g)	Fibre (g)	Pro (g)	Fat (g)
Tabasco, 1 tsp	–	–	–	–	–
Tartare sauce, 1 tbsp	77	1.3	n/a	0.1	7.9
Tomato ketchup, 1 tbsp	19	4.7	n/a	0.3	–
Wild rowan jelly, 2 tsp	27	6.5	n/a	–	–
Worcestershire sauce, 1 tsp	4	1.0	–	–	–
Mustards					
Dijon mustard, 1 tsp	5	0.1	0.1	0.3	0.4
English mustard, 1 tsp	9	0.9	0.1	0.3	0.4
French mustard, 1 tsp	7	0.6	–	0.3	0.3
Honey mustard, 1 tsp	9	1.2	0.3	0.3	0.2
Horseradish mustard, 1 tsp	8	1.2	0.2	0.3	0.2
Peppercorn mustard, 1 tsp	7	0.8	0.3	0.4	0.3
Wholegrain mustard, 1tsp:	8	0.5	0.2	0.5	0.5
hot, 1 tsp	7	0.6	0.4	0.4	0.2
Pickles and Chutneys					
Apple chutney, 1 tbsp	28	7.3	n/a	0.1	–
Barbecue relish, 1 tbsp	14	3.1	n/a	0.3	–
Chunky fruit chutney, 1 tbsp:	16	3.9	n/a	0.1	–
small chunk	21	–	0.2	0.1	–

TIP: A simple cranberry sauce can liven up fish as well as poultry. Make your own by cooking fresh cranberries with a little water over a moderate heat until they pop, then stir in a little sugar and serve warm or cold.

Condiments & Sauces	Cal (kcal)	Carb (g)	Fibre (g)	Pro (g)	Fat (g)
Chunky fruit chutney, *contd*:					
spicy	21	5.1	0.2	0.1	–
Lime pickle, 1 tbsp	29	0.6	0.1	0.3	2.8
Mango chutney, 1 tbsp	31	7.5	0.2	0.1	–
Mango with ginger chutney					
1 tbsp	28	6.9	0.1	0.1	–
Mediterranean chutney, 1 tbsp	17.9	3.9	0.2	0.3	0.1
Mustard pickle, mild, 1 tbsp	19	3.8	0.1	0.3	0.2
Piccalilli, 1 tbsp	16	3.2	0.1	0.2	0.1
Ploughman's pickle, 1 tbsp	17	4	0.1	0.1	–
Sandwich pickle, tangy, 1 tbsp	20	4.7	0.1	0.1	–
Sauerkraut, 2 tbsp	3	0.4	n/a	0.4	Tr
Spiced fruit chutney, 1 tbsp	21	5.1	n/a	0.1	–
Spreadable chutney, 1 tbsp	36	8.8	0.2	–	–
Sweet chilli dipping sauce,					
1 tbsp	33	7.8	0.1	0.1	–
Sweet pickle, 1 tbsp	21	5.4	n/a	0.1	–
Tomato chutney, 1 tbsp	19	4.6	n/a	0.2	–
Tomato pickle, tangy, 1 tbsp	25	5.2	0.4	0.5	–
Tomato with red pepper					
chutney, 1 tbsp	25	5.7	0.2	0.3	

TIP: Use a tomato salsa – a mixture of finely chopped tomatoes, coriander, red onions, lime juice and an optional chopped chilli – instead of tomato ketchup.

Condiments & Sauces	Cal (kcal)	Carb (g)	Fibre (g)	Pro (g)	Fat (g)
Salad Dressings					
Balsamic dressing, 2 tbsp	92	2.2	–	0.1	9.1
Blue cheese dressing, 2 tbsp	137	2.6	n/a	0.6	13.9
Blue cheese-flavoured low-fat dressing, 2 tbsp	18	1.8	–	0.5	1
Creamy Caesar dressing, 2 tbsp	101		–	0.9	9.6
Caesar-style low-fat dressing, 2 tbsp	24	4.4	0.1	1	0.3
Creamy low-fat salad dressing, 2 tbsp	37	4.5	n/a	0.2	2
French dressing, 2 tbsp	139	1.4	–	–	14.9
Italian dressing, 2 tbsp	36	1.7	0.1	–	3.1
fat free	10	2	0.2	–	Tr
Mayonnaise, 1 tbsp	109	0.3	–	0.2	11.9
light, reduced calorie, 1 tbsp	96	2.5	0.2	0.3	9.5
Salad cream, 1 tbsp	52	2.5	–	0.2	4.7
light, 1 tbsp	36	2	Tr	0.3	3
Seafood sauce, 1 tbsp	80	1.5	0.1	0.3	8.1
Thousand Island, 1 tbsp	55	2.9	0.1	0.1	4.7
fat free, 1 tbsp	13	3	0.4	0.1	–
Vinaigrette, 2 tbsp	139	1.4	–	–	14.8

TIP: Tabasco sauce is a good way to perk up soups, casseroles, even salad dressings. It is made from the powerful tabasco chilli pepper, so go easy; you only need a few drops to make a difference.

Condiments & Sauces	Cal (kcal)	Carb (g)	Fibre (g)	Pro (g)	Fat (g)
Vinegars					
Balsamic vinegar, 1 tbsp	15	3.2	–	Tr	–
Cider vinegar, 1 tbsp	3	0.2	–	–	–
Red wine vinegar, 1 tbsp	4	0.1	–	–	–
Sherry vinegar, 1 tbsp	4	0.3	–	0.1	–
White wine vinegar, 1 tbsp	3	0.1	–	–	–
Cooking Sauces					
Bread sauce, 100ml:					
made with semi-skimmed milk	97	15.3	n/a	4.2	2.5
made with whole milk	110	15.2	n/a	4.1	4
Cheese sauce, 100ml:					
made with semi-skimmed milk	181	8.8	n/a	8.2	12.8
made with whole milk	198	8.7	n/a	8.1	14.8
Curry sauce, canned, 100ml	78	7.1	n/a	1.5	5
Onion sauce, 100ml:					
made with semi-skimmed milk	88	8.2	n/a	3	5.1
made with whole milk	101	8.1	n/a	2.9	6.6
Pesto:					
fresh, homemade 100ml	45	6	1.4	2.2	1.3
green pesto, jar, 100ml	374	0.8	1.4	5	39

TIP: To lower the calorie count of low-fat mayonnaise further, mix it with the same quantity of no-fat Greek yoghurt. Add some chopped chives or fresh herbs, such as coriander, to make it special.

Condiments & Sauces	Cal (kcal)	Carb (g)	Fibre (g)	Pro (g)	Fat (g)
Pesto *contd:*					
red pesto, jar, 100ml	358	3.1	0.4	4.1	36.6
Tomato & basil, fresh, 100ml	51	8.8	1.3	1.8	0.9
White sauce, 100ml:					
made with semi-skimmed milk	130	10.7	n/a	4.4	8
made with whole milk	151	10.6	n/a	4.2	10.3
For more pasta sauces, *see under:* Pasta and Pizza					
Stock Cubes					
Beef, each	32	2.3	Tr	0.9	2.3
Chicken, each	32	2.3	Tr	0.9	1.8
Fish, each	32	0.5	Tr	1.8	2.3
Garlic herb & spice, each	33	5.3	0.4	1.5	0.6
Ham , each	32	1.8	Tr	1.4	1.8
Lamb, each	32	0.5	Tr	1.4	2.3
Rice saffron, each	32	1.4	0.4	1.6	2.2
Pork, each	32	1.4	Tr	1.4	2.3
Vegetable, each	45	1.4	Tr	1.4	4.1
Yeast extract, each	27	2.8	n/a	2.7	0.5

TIP: Try using low-fat natural yoghurt as a salad dressing rather than oil and vinegar. Add chopped cucumber to make tzatziki, or stir in some Dijon mustard for a spicier taste.

Dairy	Cal (kcal)	Carb (g)	Fibre (g)	Pro (g)	Fat (g)
Milk and Cream					
Buttermilk, 250ml	138	20.3	n/a	14.3	Tr
Cream:					
extra thick, 2 tbsp	70	1.1	–	0.8	6.9
fresh, clotted, 2 tbsp	176	0.7	n/a	0.5	19.1
fresh, double, 2 tbsp	149	0.5	–	0.5	16.1
fresh, single, 2 tbsp	58	0.7		1	5.7
fresh, soured, 2 tbsp	62	0.9	n/a	0.9	6.0
fresh, whipping, 2 tbsp	114	0.8	–	0.6	12
sterilised, canned, 2 tbsp	76	1.2	n/a	0.8	7.6
UHT, aerosol spray, 2 tbsp	86	2.5	–	0.6	8.3
UHT, double, vegetarian, 2 tbsp	92	1.2	0.2	0.8	9.3
UHT, single, vegetarian, 2 tbsp	44	1.4	0.1	0.9	3.9
Crème fraiche:					
full fat, 2 tbsp	113	0.7	–	0.7	12
half fat, 2 tbsp	49	1.3	–	0.8	4.5
Milk, fresh:					
cows', whole, 250ml	165	11.3	n/a	8.3	9.8
cows', semi-skimmed, 250ml	115	11.8	–	8.5	4.3
cows', skimmed, 250ml	80	11	–	8.5	0.5
cows', Channel Island, 250ml	195	12	n/a	9	12.8

TIP: Use low- or no-fat dairy products when possible but check the ingredient lists. Some low-fat products, particularly fruit yoghurts, may be high in sugar.

Dairy	Cal (kcal)	Carb (g)	Fibre (g)	Pro (g)	Fat (g)
Milk, *contd:*					
goats', pasteurised, 250ml	155	11	–	7.8	9.3
sheep's, 250ml	233	12.8	–	13.5	14.5
Milk, evaporated:					
original, 100ml	160	11.5	–	8.2	9
light, 100ml	110	10.5	–	7.5	4
Milk, dried, skimmed, 250ml	515	75.5	n/a	51.5	0.8
Milk, condensed:					
whole milk, sweetened, 100ml	333	55.5	n/a	8.5	10.1
skimmed milk, sweetened, 100ml	267	60	n/a	10	0.2
Soya milk:					
unsweetened, 250ml	65	1.3	1.3	6	4
sweetened, 250ml	108	6.3	Tr	7.8	6
Rice drink:					
calcium enriched, 250ml	125	24	–	0.3	3
vanilla, organic, 250ml	123	23.8	–	0.3	3
Yoghurt and Fromage Frais					
Diet yoghurts, 125g:					
banana	66	10.9	n/a	5.5	0.1
cherry	63	9.9	n/a	5.5	0.1
vanilla	66	10.4	n/a	5.8	0.1

TIP: Low-fat crème fraîche is stable when heated, unlike some dairy products, and is therefore great to use in cooking – in sauces, for example.

Dairy	Cal (kcal)	Carb (g)	Fibre (g)	Pro (g)	Fat (g)
Fromage frais, 1 pot (50g):					
fruit	62	7	Tr	2.7	2.8
plain	57	2.2	–	3.1	4
virtually fat free, fruit	25	2.8	0.4	3.4	0.1
virtually fat free, plain	25	2.3	–	3.9	0.1
Fruit corner, 125g:					
blueberry	140	19.4	n/a	4.6	4.9
strawberry	148	21.4	n/a	4.6	4.9
Greek-style, cows, fruit, 1 pot (125g)	171	14	Tr	6	10.5
Greek-style, cows, plain, 1 pot (125g)	166	6	–	7.1	12.8
Greek-style, sheep, 1 pot (125g)	115	6.3	–	6	7.5
Low fat, fruit, 1 pot (125g)	98	17.1	0.4	5.3	1.4
Low fat, plain, 1 pot (125g)	70	9.3	–	6	1.3
Natural bio yoghurt, 125g	68	7	–	5.5	1.9
Orange fat-free bio yoghurt each	61	11.3	0.1	5.4	0.2
Raspberry drinking yoghurt, per bottle	78	12.5	0.1	2.9	1.8
Soya, fruit, 1 pot (125g)	91	16.1	0.9	2.6	2.25
Virtually fat free, fruit, 1 pot (125g)	59	8.78	Tr	6	0.3

TIP: Opt for strong-flavoured cheese to add to recipes so that you will need less to get the taste you want.

Dairy	Cal (kcal)	Carb (g)	Fibre (g)	Pro (g)	Fat (g)
Virtually fat free, plain, 1 pot					
(125g)	68	10.3	–	6.8	0.3
Yoghurt drink, 125ml:					
natural	84	8.6	n/a	6.9	2.4
peach	94	16.2	n/a	3.2	1.8
Whole milk, fruit, 1 pot (125g)	136	22.1	–	5	3.8
Whole milk, plain, 1 pot (125g)	99	9.8	–	7.1	3.8
Butter and Margarine					
Butter:					
lightly salted, 15g	111	–	n/a	–	12.2
spreadable, 15g	112	Tr	–	0.1	12.4
lighter spreadable, 15g	82	0.1	–	0.1	9
Margarine, hard					
animal & vegetable fat,					
over 80% fat, 15g	108	0.2	n/a	–	11.9
Margarine, soft					
polyunsaturated, over 80%					
fat, 15g	112	–	n/a	Tr	12.4
Spreads					
Olive oil spread, 15g	80	0.2	Tr	–	8.9

TIP: Mix fruit purée with no- or low-fat Greek yoghurt for a quick fruit fool without the calorie load of double cream.

Dairy	Cal (kcal)	Carb (g)	Fibre (g)	Pro (g)	Fat (g)
Olive oil spread, *contd*:					
very low fat (20-25%)	39	0.4	–	0.9	3.8
Polyunsaturated spread:					
buttery, 15g	80	–	–	Tr	8.9
light, 15g	55	0.9	–	–	5.7
low salt, 15g	80	Tr	–	Tr	8.9
sunflower spread, 15g	95	–	–	–	10.5
Pro-biotic, 15g	50	0.6	Tr	–	5.3
light	34	0.2	Tr	0.5	3.5
Cheeses					
Bel Paese, individual, 25g	77	–	–	5.8	6
Bavarian smoked, 25g	69	0.1	–	4.3	5.8
Brie, 25g	76	0.1	–	5.5	6
Caerphilly, 25g	93	–	–	5.8	7.8
Cambozola, 25g	108	0.1	–	3.3	10.5
Camembert, 25g	73	Tr	–	5.4	5.7
Cheddar:					
English, 25g	104	–	–	6.4	8.7
vegetarian, 25g	98	Tr	–	6.4	8
Cheddar-type, half fat, 25g	68	Tr	–	8.2	4

TIP: Don't add butter to spinach. Mix cooked spinach with a little low-fat natural yoghurt instead, then sprinkle with some black pepper and, if you like the taste, a little grated nutmeg.

Dairy	Cal (kcal)	Carb (g)	Fibre (g)	Pro (g)	Fat (g)
Cheshire, 25g	93	–	–	5.8	7.8
Cottage cheese:					
plain, 100g	101	3.1	–	12.6	4.3
reduced fat, 100g	79	3.3	–	13.3	1.5
with additions, 100g	95	2.6	–	12.8	3.8
Cream cheese, full fat, 25g	110	Tr	n/a	0.8	11.9
ail & fines herbs, 25g	104	0.5	–	1.8	10.5
au naturel, 25g	106	0.5	–	1.8	10.8
au poivre, 25g	104	0.5	–	1.8	10.5
Danish Blue, 25g	86	Tr	–	5.1	7.2
Dolcelatte, 25g	99	0.2	–	4.3	9
Double Gloucester, 25g	101	–	–	6	8.5
Edam, 25g	85	Tr	–	6.7	6.5
Emmenthal, 25g	93	0.1	–	7.3	7
Feta, 25g	63	0.4	–	3.9	5.1
Goats' milk soft cheese, 25g	80	0.3	–	5.3	6.5
Gorgonzola, 25g	78	–	–	4.8	6.5
Gouda, 25g	94	Tr	–	6.3	7.7
Grana Padano, 25g	98	–	–	8.8	7
Gruyère, 25g	99	–	–	6.8	8
Jarlsberg, 25g	91	–	–	7	7
Lancashire, 25g	93	–	–	5.8	7.8

TIP: Make lassi by beating low-fat natural yoghurt until frothy then diluting it with water. Garnish with a few mint leaves.

Dairy	Cal (kcal)	Carb (g)	Fibre (g)	Pro (g)	Fat (g)
Mascarpone, 25g	104	1.2	–	1.2	10.5
Mature cheese, reduced fat, 25g	77	–	–	6.8	5.5
Medium-fat soft cheese, 25g	50	0.9	–	2.5	4.1
Mild cheese, reduced fat, 25g	77	–	–	6.8	5.5
Mozzarella, 25g	64	–	–	4.7	5.1
Parmesan, fresh, 25g	104	0.2	–	9.1	7.4
Quark, 25g	15	1	–	2.8	0.1
Red Leicester, 25g	101	–	–	6	8.5
Ricotta, 25g	34	0.5	–	2.3	2.5
Roquefort, 25g	89	Tr	–	5.8	7.3
Sage Derby, 25g	104	0.7	–	6.1	8.5
Shropshire blue, 25g	92	0.1	–	5.5	7.8
Soft cheese:					
full fat, 25g	63	0.8	0.1	1.5	6
light medium fat, 25g	47	0.9	0.1	2	3.9
light with chives, 25g	46	0.9	0.1	1.9	3.9
light with tomato & basil, 25g	45	1.1	0.1	1.9	3.5
Stilton:					
blue, 25g	103	–	–	5.9	8.8
white, 25g	90	–	–	5	7.8
white, with apricots, 25g	8	2	0.4	4	6.3
Wensleydale, 25g	95	–	–	5.8	8

TIP: Soya milk is derived from soya beans and retains most of their nutritional value. Choose unsweetened soya milk fortified with calcium.

Dairy	Cal (kcal)	Carb (g)	Fibre (g)	Pro (g)	Fat (g)
Wensleydale, *contd:*					
with cranberries, 25g	91	2.3	–	5.3	6.8
Cheese Spreads and Processed Cheese					
Cheese spread:					
original, 25g	62	0.9	0.1	3.5	5
cheese & chive, 25g	59	1	0.1	3.1	4.8
cheese & shrimp, 25g	59	0.7	0.1	3.6	4.6
cheese & ham, 25g	60	0.9	0.1	3.3	4.8
cheese & garlic, 25g	62	1	–	3.9	5
light, 25g	43	1.7	–	4	5
Cheese slices:					
singles, 25g	65	1.9	0.1	3.4	3.6
singles light, 25g	51	1.5	–	5	2.8
Cheese triangles, 25g	60	1.5	–	2.6	4.9
Processed cheese, plain, 25g	74	1.3	–	4.5	5.8
Strip cheese, 25g	88	0.3	–	5.4	6.9

TIP: A 25g portion of cheeses, as listed in this section, is a piece about the size of three stacked dice, or the size of your thumb. Sliced or grated, it would be just enough for a modest cheese sandwich. Don't get carried away – check the calorie and fat counts for your favourites.

Desserts & Puddings	Cal (kcal)	Carb (g)	Fibre (g)	Pro (g)	Fat (g)
Puddings					
Bread pudding, 100g	289	48	n/a	5.9	9.5
Christmas pudding, 100g	329	56.3	n/a	3	11.8
Creamed rice, 100g	93	16	Tr	3.2	2.9
Meringue, 100g	381	96	n/a	5.3	Tr
Pavlova, with raspberries, 100g	297	45	Tr	2.5	11.9
Profiteroles, 100g	358	18.5	0.4	6.2	29.2
Rice pudding, 100g:	130	19.6	0.1	4.1	4.3
with sultanas & nutmeg	105	16.6	0.1	3.2	2.9
Sago pudding, 100g:					
made with semi-skimmed milk	93	20.1	0.1	4	0.2
made with whole milk	130	19.6	0.1	4.1	4.3
Semolina pudding, 100g:					
made with semi-skimmed milk	93	20.1	0.1	4	0.2
made with whole milk	130	19.6	0.1	4.1	4.3
Sponge pudding:					
with chocolate sauce, 100g	303	44.6	1.2	5.2	11.5
lemon, 100g	306	50.1	0.6	2.7	10.6
treacle, 100g	286	50	0.6	2.6	8.4
Spotted Dick, 100g	337	52.7	1	3.4	12.6
Tapioca pudding, 100g:					
made with semi-skimmed milk	93	20.1	0.1	4	0.2

TIP: A platter of beautifully arranged, perfectly ripe, fresh fruit scattered with a few nuts makes an excellent finale to a meal.

Desserts & Puddings	Cal (kcal)	Carb (g)	Fibre (g)	Pro (g)	Fat (g)
Tapioca pudding, 100g, *contd:*					
made with whole milk	130	19.6	0.1	4.1	4.3
Trifle, 100g	166	21	Tr	2.6	8.1
Trifle with fresh cream, 100g	166	19.5	0.5	2.4	9.2
Sweet Pies and Flans					
Apple & blackcurrant pies, each	227	35.7	1	2.3	8.4
Apple pie, 100g	384	57.8	1.2	3.2	15.5
Bakewell tart, 100g	397	56.7	0.9	3.8	17.2
cherry bakewell, each	199	28.4	0.7	1.8	8.7
Cheesecake, 100g:	294	35.2	1	4	16.2
raspberry	299	31.9	0.6	4.7	17.2
Custard tart, 100g	277	32.4	–	6.3	14.5
Dutch apple tart, 100g	237	34.4	0.6	3.2	9.9
Fruit pie, individual:	356	56.7	–	4.3	14
pastry top & bottom, 100g	262	33.9	n/a	3.1	13.6
wholemeal, one crust, 100g	185	26.5	n/a	2.7	8.3
Jam tart, each	139	22.4	0.5	1.3	4.9
Lemon meringue pie, 100g	251	43.5	–	2.9	8.5
Mince pies, 100g	395	59.9	1.5	3.7	15.6
luxury, 100g	387	55.7	1.5	3.7	14
Treacle tart, 100g	379	62.8	n/a	3.9	14.2

TIP: Push fresh raspberries through a sieve to make a raspberry purée. Spoon over vanilla ice cream, and top with whole fresh raspberries.

Desserts & Puddings	Cal (kcal)	Carb (g)	Fibre (g)	Pro (g)	Fat (g)
Chilled and Frozen Desserts					
Crème brulée, 100g	251	23.5	0.2	1.3	17
Crème caramel, 100g	104	20.6	n/a	3	1.6
Chocolate nut sundae, 100g	243	26.2	0.2	2.6	14.9
Ice cream, 100g:					
Cornish	92	11.3	n/a	19	4.4
chocolate	91	11.4	n/a	2	4.2
Neapolitan	83	11.8	Tr	1.7	3.3
peach melba	94	13.2	n/a	1.7	3.8
raspberry ripple	87	13.1	Tr	1.6	3.1
strawberry	84	10.5	n/a	1.7	3.8
tiramisu	112	15.2	n/a	2.1	4.6
vanilla	87	11.0	n/a	1.7	4.5
Ice cream bar, chocolate-covered, 100g	311	21.8	Tr	5	23.3
Ice cream dessert, frozen, 100g	251	21	Tr	3.5	17.6
Instant dessert powder, 100g:					
made up with whole milk	111	14.8	0.2	3.1	6.3
Jelly, 100g, made with water	296	68.9	n/a	5.1	–
Mousse, 100g:					
chocolate	149	19.9	–	4	6.5
fruit	143	18	–	4.5	6.4

TIP: Toast chopped almonds in a dry frying pan and stir them into no-fat Greek yoghurt. Drizzle a little runny honey over the top.

Desserts & Puddings	Cal (kcal)	Carb (g)	Fibre (g)	Pro (g)	Fat (g)
Sorbet, 100g:					
fruit	97	24.8	1	0.2	0.3
lemon	128	32	–	–	–
Tiramisu, 100g	337	31.2	0.3	3.5	22.2
Vanilla soya dessert, each	80	16.4	1.3	3.8	2.3
For yoghurt, *see under Dairy*					
Toppings and Sauces					
Brandy sauce, ready to serve, 50ml	49	8.3	–	1.4	0.8
Chocolate custard mix, 50ml:	208	39.3	0.1	3.0	4.4
Custard, 50ml:					
made with skimmed milk	40	8.4	Tr	1.9	0.1
made with whole milk	59	8.1	n/a	2	2.3
canned or carton	50	7	Tr	1.5	2
Devon custard, canned, 50ml	51	8	–	1.5	1.5
Artificial cream topping, 50ml	345	16.3	0.3	3.4	29.3
sugar-free	348	15.3	0.3	3.7	30.3
Maple syrup, organic, 1 tsp	17	4.2	Tr	Tr	–

TIP: When it comes to ice cream, the taste of a gourmet brand will be light years better than the supermarket's own-brand economy pack. If you're eating smaller portions, maybe you can afford to splash out.

Drinks	Cal (kcal)	Carb (g)	Fibre (g)	Pro (g)	Fat (g)
Alcoholic					
Advocaat, 25ml	68	7.1	–	1.2	1.6
Beer, bitter:					
canned, 500ml	160	11.5	–	1.5	Tr
draught, 1 pint	182	13	–	1.7	Tr
keg, 1 pint	176	13	–	1.7	Tr
Beer, mild draught, 1 pint	142	9.1	–	1.1	Tr
Brandy, 25ml	56	Tr	–	Tr	–
Brown ale, bottled, 500ml	150	15	n/a	1.5	–
Cider, 500ml:					
dry	180	13	n/a	Tr	–
sweet	210	21.5	n/a	Tr	–
vintage	505	36.5	n/a	Tr	–
Cognac, 25ml	88	n/a	n/a	n/a	n/a
Gin, 25ml	56	Tr	–	Tr	–
Lager, bottled, 500ml	145	7.5	–	1.0	Tr
Pale ale, bottled, 500ml	140	10	n/a	1.5	Tr
Port, 25ml	39	3	n/a	–	–
Rum, 25ml	56	Tr	–	Tr	–
Sherry, 25ml					
dry	29	0.4	n/a	0.1	–
medium	29	1.5	n/a	–	–

TIP: One pint of beer is equivalent to 568ml. A 500ml botle or tin contains less than 1 pint.

Drinks	Cal (kcal)	Carb (g)	Fibre (g)	Pro (g)	Fat (g)
Sherry, *contd*					
sweet	34	1.7	n/a	0.1	–
Stout, 500ml:					
bottled	185	21	–	1.5	Tr
extra	195	10.5	–	1.5	Tr
Strong ale, 500ml	360	30.5	–	3.5	Tr
Vermouth, 50ml:					
dry	55	1.5	n/a	0.1	–
sweet	76	8.0	n/a	Tr	–
bianco	73	n/a	n/a	n/a–	n/a
extra dry	48	n/a	n/a	n/a	n/a
rosso	70	n/a	n/a	n/a	n/a
Vodka, 25ml	56	Tr	–	Tr	–
Whisky, 25ml	56	Tr	–	Tr	–
Wine, per small glass (125ml):					
red	85	0.3	n/a	0.1	–
rosé	89	3.1	n/a	0.1	–
white, dry	83	0.8	n/a	0.1	–
white, medium	93	3.8	n/a	0.1	–
white, sparkling	93	6.4	n/a	0.4	–
white, sweet	118	7.4	n/a	0.3	–

TIP: Alcohol contains 'empty' calories and can slow down your body's consumption of fat – while your system has alcohol as a source of energy it won't use up other sources, such as body fat.

Drinks	Cal (kcal)	Carb (g)	Fibre (g)	Pro (g)	Fat (g)
Liqueurs					
Cherry, 25ml	64	8.2	–	Tr	–
Coffee, 25ml	65.5	n/a	n/a	n/a	–
Coffee cream, 25ml	80	n/a	n/a	n/a	–
Orange, 25ml	85	n/a	n/a	n/a	–
Triple sec, 25ml	80	n/a	n/a	n/a	–
Juices and Cordials					
Apple juice,					
unsweetened, 250ml	95	24.8	n/a	0.3	0.3
Apple & elderflower juice,					
250ml	108	25.5	n/a	1	0.3
Apple & mango juice, 250ml	108	25.3	n/a	1	0.3
Barley water, 250ml:					
lemon, original	241	54.5	Tr	0.8	Tr
no added sugar	28	27.5	–	0.5	–
orange, original	244	57.8	Tr	0.8	Tr
Blackcurrant & apple juice,					
250ml	108	24.3	n/a	Tr	Tr
Carrot juice, 250ml	60	14.3	–	1.3	0.3
Cranberry juice, 250ml	123	29.3	Tr	Tr	Tr

TIP: Iced tea makes a refreshing summer drink. Make a pot of good tea, or use herb tea, then strain and chill for an hour. Serve in tall glasses over crushed ice with a slice of lemon and a sprig of mint.

Drinks	Cal (kcal)	Carb (g)	Fibre (g)	Pro (g)	Fat (g)
Grape juice, unsweetened, 250ml	115	29.3	–	0.8	0.3
Grapefruit juice, 250ml	103	22	n/a	1.3	Tr
Lemon squash, low calorie, 250ml	18	1	n/a	–	–
Lime juice cordial, undiluted, 25ml	28	7.5	n/a	–	–
Orange & mango fruit juice, no added sugar, 250ml	21	2	n/a	0.5	Tr
Orange & pineapple fruit juice, 250ml	120	27.5	n/a	1.3	Tr
Orange juice, unsweetened, 250ml	90	22	n/a	1.3	0.3
Orange squash, low calorie, 250ml	25	6	–	0.3	–
Pineapple juice, unsweetened, 250ml	103	26.3	n/a	0.8	0.3
Tomato juice, 250ml:	35	7.5	n/a	2	Tr
cocktail (Britvic), 250ml	52	9	n/a	2.3	0.3

TIP: If you want to cut down on the amount of alcohol you drink, start keeping a diary of the number of units you consume. A unit is a small pub measure of wine (125ml), one unit of spirits (25ml) or a half pint (284ml) of lager. Remember that government-recommended totals are 14 units a week for women and 21 a week for men.

Drinks	Cal (kcal)	Carb (g)	Fibre (g)	Pro (g)	Fat (g)
Fizzy Drinks					
Apple drink, sparkling, 330ml	95	22.4	n/a	Tr	Tr
Bitter lemon, 355ml	126	29.5	n/a	Tr	Tr
Cherry Coke, 330ml	149	36.3	n/a	–	–
Cherryade, 330ml	94	22.4	n/a	Tr	Tr
Cola, 330ml	142	35	n/a	–	–
diet	1	–	n/a	–	–
Cream Soda, 330ml	71	17.5	n/a	–	–
Dandelion & Burdock, 330ml	65	16.2	n/a	Tr	Tr
Ginger Ale, American 330ml	124	30.4	n/a	–	–
Ginger Ale, Dry 330ml	52	12.5	n/a	–	–
Ginger beer, 330ml	116	28.1	n/a	Tr	–
Irn Bru, 330ml	135	33.3	–	Tr	Tr
diet, 330ml	2	Tr	–	Tr	Tr
Lemon drink, sparkling, 330ml	165	39.6	n/a	–	–
low calorie	7	1.3	n/a	–	–
Lemonade, 330ml	73	19.1	n/a	Tr	–
low calorie	5	Tr	n/a	Tr	Tr
Glucose drink, 330ml	241	59.1	n/a	Tr	–
Orange drink, 330ml	96	22.1	n/a	Tr	Tr
low calorie	18	2.3	n/a	Tr	Tr

TIP: Remember that caffeine can play havoc with your insulin levels. It isn't only found in coffee and tea – cola drinks, including diet colas, are very high in it too.

Drinks	Cal (kcal)	Carb (g)	Fibre (g)	Pro (g)	Fat (g)
Ribena, sparkling, 330ml	178	43.9	–	–	–
low calorie	7	0.3	–	–	–
Tonic water, 330ml	86	20.5	n/a	–	–
Water, flavoured, 330ml	3	Tr	–	Tr	–
Hot and Milky Drinks					
Beef instant drink, per mug	425	51.3	0.3	54.3	0.3
Cappuccino, per sachet:					
instant	72	12	–	2	1.7
unsweetened	77	9.8	–	2.7	3
Chicken instant drink, per mug	323	48.8	5.3	24.3	3.5
Cocoa, per mug					
made with semi-skimmed milk	142	17.4	0.5	8.7	4.7
made with whole milk	190	17.0	0.5	8.5	10.5
Coffee, black, per mug	5	0.8	n/a	0.5	Tr
Coffee creamer, per tsp	26	3.7	–	0.2	2.2
virtually fat free, per tsp	20	4.2	–	0.1	0.3
Drinking chocolate, per mug					
made with semi-skimmed milk	183	27.3	–	9	5
made with whole milk	225	26.8	2.5	8.8	10
Espresso, per 100ml	104	10	11.5	15.2	0.4

TIP: If you know that you'll find restricting the amount of alcohol you drink difficult, then it's best to cut it out completely as you diet down to your target weight. The weight will drop off much faster.

Drinks	Cal (kcal)	Carb (g)	Fibre (g)	Pro (g)	Fat (g)
Herb teas, per mug	–	–	–	0.1	–
Ice tea, per mug	70	16.8	n/a	–	–
Malted milk, per mug					
made with semi-skimmed milk	460	71.3	1.8	23.5	11.5
made with whole milk	575	70.8	1.8	23	22.8
Malted milk light,					
made with water, per mug	290	57.8	1.5	11.8	3.0
Strawberry milkshake, 250ml					
made with semi-skimmed milk	387	62.2	–	17	8.5
made with whole milk	420	47.2	–	17	19.5
Tea, black, per cup	Tr	Tr	n/a	0.3	Tr

TIP: A tablespoon or so of a liqueur like Grand Marnier or Cointreau on a fruit salad can give it a delicious flavour and avoid the need to use fruit syrups or juices.

Fish & Seafood	Cal (kcal)	Carb (g)	Fibre (g)	Pro (g)	Fat (g)
Fish and Seafood					
Anchovies, in oil,					
drained, 100g	191	–	–	25.2	10
Cockles, boiled, 100g	53	Tr	n/a	12	0.6
Cod:					
baked fillets, 100g	96	Tr	n/a	21.4	1.2
dried, salted, boiled, 100g	138	–	n/a	32.5	0.9
in batter, fried, 100g	247	11.7	n/a	16.1	15.4
in crumbs, fried, 100g	235	15.2	n/a	12.4	14.3
in parsley sauce, boiled, 100g	84	2.8	n/a	12	2.8
poached fillets, 100g	94	Tr	n/a	20.9	1.1
steaks, grilled, 100g	95	Tr	n/a	20.8	1.3
Cod roe, hard, fried, 100g	202	3	n/a	20.9	11.9
Coley fillets, steamed, 100g	105	–	n/a	23.3	1.3
Crab					
boiled, 100g	128	Tr	n/a	19.5	5.5
canned, 100g	77	Tr	n/a	18.1	0.5
dressed, 100g	105	n/a	n/a	16.9	14.2
Eels, jellied, 100g	98	Tr	n/a	8.4	7.1
Haddock:					
in crumbs, fried, 100g	196	12.6	n/a	14.7	10

TIP: Tinned tuna is a useful storecupboard standby. Always buy it in brine or spring water, and rinse before use to reduce salt levels. For a tasty tuna dip, blend it with low-fat cream cheese and a little paprika.

Fish & Seafood	Cal (kcal)	Carb (g)	Fibre (g)	Pro (g)	Fat (g)
Haddock, *contd*:					
smoked, steamed, 100g	101	–	n/a	23.3	0.9
steamed, 100g	89	–	n/a	20.9	0.6
Halibut, grilled, 100g	121	–	n/a	25.3	2.2
Herring:					
fried, 100g	234	1.5	–	23.1	15.1
grilled, 100g	199	–	–	20.4	13
Kippers, grilled, 100g	255	–	n/a	20.1	19.4
Lemon sole:					
steamed, 100g	91	–	n/a	20.6	0.9
goujons, baked, 100g	187	14.7	n/a	16	14.6
goujons, fried, 100g	374	14.3	n/a	15.5	28.7
Lobster, boiled, 100g	119	–	–	22.1	3.4
Mackerel, grilled, 100g	239	–	n/a	20.8	17.3
Mussels, boiled, 100g	87	Tr	–	17.2	2
Pilchards,					
canned in tomato sauce, 100g	126	0.7	Tr	18.8	5.4
Plaice					
in batter, fried, 100g	257	12	–	15.2	16.8
in crumbs, fried, 100g	228	8.6	–	18	13.7
goujons, baked, 100g	304	27.7	–	8.8	18.3

TIP: Don't serve a rich hollandaise sauce with salmon. Instead try finely chopped cucumber or spring onion, mixed with equal measures of no-fat Greek yoghurt and low-fat mayo.

Fish & Seafood	Cal (kcal)	Carb (g)	Fibre (g)	Pro (g)	Fat (g)
Plaice, *contd*:					
goujons, fried, 100g	426	27	–	8.5	32.3
steamed, 100g	93	–	–	18.9	1.9
Prawns: *shelled, boiled*, 100g	99	–	n/a	22.6	0.9
boiled, weighed in shells, 175g	72	–	–	15.1	1.2
king prawns, freshwater, 100g	70	–	n/a	16.8	0.3
North Atlantic, peeled, 100g	99	–	–	22.6	0.9
tiger king, cooked, 100g	61	–	n/a	13.5	0.6
Roe:					
cod, hard, fried, 100g	202	3	n/a	20.9	11.9
herring, soft, fried, 100g	244	4.7	–	21.1	15.8
Salmon:					
pink, canned in brine, drained, 100g	153	–	n/a	23.5	6.6
grilled steak, 100g	215	–	n/a	24.2	13.1
smoked, 100g	142	–	n/a	25.4	4.5
steamed, flesh only, 100g	194	–	n/a	21.8	11.9
Sardines:					
canned in oil, drained, 100g	220	–	n/a	23.3	14.1
canned in tomato sauce, 100g	162	1.4	n/a	17	9.9
Scampi tails, premium, 100g	230	26	n/a	8.4	10.9

TIP: Anchovies are one of the oily fishes, related to herrings. Always drain them of their oil and blot dry on kitchen paper before use. They can add a useful burst of flavour to a salad or dressing.

Fish & Seafood	Cal (kcal)	Carb (g)	Fibre (g)	Pro (g)	Fat (g)
Shrimps:					
canned, drained, 100g	94	Tr	n/a	20.8	1.2
frozen, without shells, 100g	73	Tr	n/a	16.5	0.8
Skate, fried in butter, 100g	199	4.9	0.2	17.9	12.1
Sole: *see* Lemon sole					
Swordfish, grilled, 100g	139	–	n/a	22.9	5.2
Trout:					
brown, steamed, 100g	135	–	–	23.5	4.5
rainbow, grilled, 100g	135	–	n/a	21.5	5.4
Tuna, fresh, grilled, 100g	170	0.4	–	24.3	7.9
canned in brine, 100g	99	–	n/a	23.5	0.6
canned in oil, 100g	189	–	n/a	27.1	9
Whelks, boiled,					
weighed with shells, 100g	89	Tr	n/a	19.5	1.2
Whitebait, fried, 100g	525	5.3	n/a	19.5	47.5
Whiting:					
steamed, flesh only, 100g	92	–	n/a	20.9	0.9
in crumbs, fried, 100g	191	7	n/a	18.1	10.3
Winkles, boiled,					
weighed with shells, 100g	72	Tr	n/a	15.4	1.2

TIP: Fish cooks much more quickly than most meats, making it an excellent choice for anyone in a hurry; in fact, overcooking spoils it. Grill fish, or poach it in skimmed milk flavoured with a bay leaf and a little lemon rind; don't be tempted to fry it when you're dieting.

Fish & Seafood	Cal (kcal)	Carb (g)	Fibre (g)	Pro (g)	Fat (g)
Breaded, Battered or in Sauces					
Calamari in batter, 100g	177	13	1.5	7.8	10.4
Fish cakes, 100g					
fried, each	218	16.8	n/a	8.6	13.4
Fish fingers					
fried in oil, 100g	233	17.2	0.6	13.5	12.7
grilled, 100g	214	19.3	0.7	15.1	9
oven crispy, 100g	236	17	0.5	10.5	14
Fish steaks in butter sauce, 100g	84	3.2	0.1	9.1	3.9
Fish steaks in parsley sauce, 100g	82	3.1	0.1	9.1	3.7
Kipper fillets with butter, 100g	205	–	–	15	16
Prawn Cocktail (Lyons), 100g	429	4.5	n/a	5.7	42.9
Seafood sticks, 100g	95	14.5	1	8.1	0.4
Shrimps, potted, 100g	358	–	–	16.5	32.4

TIP: Fruit and fish can complement each other very successfully. Pink grapefruit and smoked salmon go well, mango works beautifully with smoked fish, and an anchovy and melon salad makes an unusual starter. Cut the melon into cubes, and chop the well-drained anchovies (soak them in milk for a while if they seem too salty). Combine and sprinkle with a little orange and lemon juice.

Fruit	Cal (kcal)	Carb (g)	Fibre (g)	Pro (g)	Fat (g)
Apple, 1 medium	82	20.4	n/a	0.7	0.2
Apples, stewed					
with sugar (60g)	44	11.5	n/a	0.2	0.1
without sugar (60g)	20	4.9	n/a	0.2	0.1
Apricots: 1 fresh	16	3.7	n/a	0.5	0.1
dried, 8 halves	45	9.9	1.7	1.1	0.2
canned in juice, 100g	34	8.4	n/a	0.5	0.1
canned in syrup, 100g	63	16.1	n/a	0.4	0.1
Avocado, half medium	160	1.6	n/a	1.6	16.4
Banana, 1 medium	95	23.2	n/a	1.2	0.3
Blackberries:					
fresh, 75g	19	3.8	n/a	0.7	0.2
stewed with sugar, 75g	42	10.4	n/a	0.5	0.2
stewed without sugar, 75g	16	3.3	4.2	0.6	0.2
Blackcurrants:					
fresh, 75g	21	5	n/a	0.7	Tr
stewed with sugar, 75g	44	11.3	n/a	0.5	Tr
canned in syrup, 75g	54	13.8	2.7	0.5	Tr
Blueberries, fresh, 75g	32	7.6	1.6	0.4	0.2
Cherries, half cup fresh (90g)	43	10.4	0.8	0.8	0.09
Cherries, glacé, 25g	63	16.6	0.2	0.1	–

TIP: If you can, buy unwaxed organic lemons, as pesticide residues can easily penetrate the skin of citrus fruit.

Fruit	Cal (kcal)	Carb (g)	Fibre (g)	Pro (g)	Fat (g)
Clementines, 1 medium	28	6.6	0.9	0.7	0.1
Coconut:					
creamed, 2 tbsp	134	1.4	n/a	1.2	13.8
desiccated, 2 tbsp	121	1.3	n/a	1.1	12.4
milk, 100ml	166	1.6	–	1.6	17.0
Cranberries, fresh, 75g	12	3	3.2	–	–
Damsons:					
fresh, 75g	29	7.2	n/a	0.4	Tr
stewed with sugar (2 tbsp)	22	5.7	n/a	0.1	Tr
Dates, quarter cup (50g)	62	15.7	n/a	0.8	0.1
Figs:					
1 fresh	37	9.6	1.7	0.4	0.2
dried, ready to eat, 50g	112	24.5	0.8	1.7	0.8
canned in syrup, 100g	75	18	0.7	0.4	0.1
Fruit cocktail, 100g					
canned in juice	29	7.2	n/a	0.4	Tr
canned in syrup	57	14.8	n/a	0.4	Tr
Gooseberries:					
fresh, 75g	14	2.3	n/a	0.8	0.3
stewed with sugar (2 tbsp)	16	3.9	n/a	0.2	0.1
Grapefruit, half, fresh	34	7.7	n/a	0.9	0.1

TIP: Make an attractive fruit salad using cubed watermelon, black seedless grapes, a little Grand Marnier and a squeeze of lemon juice. Chill for an hour before serving, stirring occasionally during this time.

Fruit	Cal (kcal)	Carb (g)	Fibre (g)	Pro (g)	Fat (g)
Grapes, black/white, seedless,					
fresh, 75g	45	11.6	n/a	0.3	0.1
Greengages:					
fresh, 75g	26	6.5	1.2	0.4	Tr
stewed with sugar (2 tbsp)	32	8	0.4	0.4	–
Guavas, fresh, 60g	16	3	n/a	0.5	0.3
Honeydew melon: see Melon					
Jackfruit, fresh, 75g	66	16.1	–	1.0	0.2
Kiwi fruit, peeled, each	49	10.6	n/a	1.1	0.5
Lemon, whole	19	3.2	n/a	1	0.3
Lychees, fresh, 75g	44	10.7	n/a	0.7	0.1
canned in syrup, 100g	68	17.7	n/a	0.4	Tr
Mandarin oranges, 100g:					
canned in juice	32	7.7	n/a	0.7	Tr
canned in syrup	52	13.4	n/a	0.5	Tr
Mangos, 1 medium	66	16.3	n/a	0.8	0.2
Melon, fresh, medium slice:					
cantaloupe	22	4.9	n/a	0.7	0.1
galia	27	6.3	n/a	0.6	0.1
honeydew	32	7.5	n/a	0.7	0.1
watermelon	35	8	n/a	0.6	0.3

TIP: Berries have very little carbohydrate and are high in fibre.
Blackcurrants and strawberries are excellent sources of vitamin C.

Fruit	Cal (kcal)	Carb (g)	Fibre (g)	Pro (g)	Fat (g)
Nectarines, 1 medium	60	13.5	n/a	2.1	0.1
Oranges, 1 medium	56	12.9	n/a	1.7	0.2
Papaya, half, fresh	41	10	n/a	0.6	0.1
Passionfruit, 75g					
fresh (flesh & pips only)	27	4.4	n/a	2	0.3
Paw-paw, half, fresh	41	10	2.5	0.6	0.1
Peach, 1 medium	50	11.5	n/a	1.5	0.2
canned in juice, 100g	39	9.7	n/a	0.6	Tr
canned in syrup, 100g	55	14	n/a	0.5	Tr
Pear, 1 medium	60	15	n/a	0.5	0.2
canned in juice, 100g	33	8.5	n/a	0.3	Tr
canned in syrup, 100g	50	13.2	n/a	0.2	Tr
Pineapple, fresh, 60g	25	6.1	n/a	0.2	0.1
canned in juice, 100g	47	12.2	n/a	0.3	Tr
canned in syrup, 100g	64	16.5	n/a	0.5	Tr
Plums, 1 medium	36	8.8	n/a	0.6	0.1
Prunes, canned in juice, 100g	79	19.7	n/a	0.7	0.2
canned in syrup, 100g	90	23	n/a	0.6	0.2
Prunes, dried: *see under* Snacks					
Raisins: *see under* Snacks					
Raspberries, fresh, 60g	15	2.8	n/a	0.8	0.2

TIP: Oranges are high in vitamin C, but are also rich in vitamins A, B1 and folic acid. Don't be tempted just to drink the juice as you'd miss out on useful fibre.

Fruit	Cal (kcal)	Carb (g)	Fibre (g)	Pro (g)	Fat (g)
Rhubarb, fresh, raw, 60g	4	0.5	n/a	0.5	0.1
stewed with sugar (2 tbsp)	14	3.4	n/a	0.3	–
stewed without sugar (2 tbsp)	2	0.2	0.4	0.3	–
Satsumas, 1 medium	54	12.8	n/a	1.4	0.2
Strawberries, 70g	19	4.2	n/a	0.6	0.1
Tangerines, fresh, one	35	8	n/a	0.9	0.1
Watermelon, see under Melon					

TIP: For a delicious fruit salad try a mix of black- and redcurrants in Cointreau. Mix 2 tablespoons Cointreau with some grated orange rind, a squeeze of orange juice and a teaspoon of honey. Put 250g each of black- and redcurrants in a serving bowl and pour the Cointreau mixture over; stir well but gently. Chill in the fridge overnight.

Jams & Spreads	Cal (kcal)	Carb (g)	Fibre (g)	Pro (g)	Fat (g)
Jams and Marmalades					
Apricot conserve, 1 tsp	13	3.2	–	–	–
Apricot fruit spread, 1 tsp:					
diet	6	1.5	–	–	–
organic	7	1.7	0.1	–	Tr
Apricot jam, 1 tsp:					
reduced sugar	9	2.3	n/a	–	–
sucrose free	13	3.2	n/a	–	Tr
Blackcurrant jam, 1 tsp:					
reduced sugar	9	2.3	n/a	–	–
sucrose free	13	3.4	n/a	–	Tr
Blueberry & blackberry jam,			–	–	–
organic, 1 tsp	13	3	0.1	–	–
Grapefruit fruit spread, 1 tsp	7	1.9	0.1	–	–
Grapefruit marmalade, 1 tsp	12	3.1	n/a	–	–
Honey, 1 tsp:					
clear	15	3.7	n/a	–	Tr
honeycomb	14	3.6	n/a	–	0.2
set	14	3.5	–	–	–
Lemon curd, 1 tsp	14	3.1	–	–	0.2
Marmalade:					
orange, 1 tsp	8	2.1	n/a	–	–

TIP: Stone some black olives and whizz them in a blender or food processor to make a tapenade – delicious spread on oatcakes.

Jams & Spreads	Cal (kcal)	Carb (g)	Fibre (g)	Pro (g)	Fat (g)
Marmalade, *contd:*					
Dundee, 1 tsp	11	2.7	–	–	–
organic, 1 tsp	13	3.2	–	–	–
thick-cut, 1 tsp	13	3.5	–	–	–
Morello cherry fruit spread					
organic, 1 tsp	7	1.7	0.1	–	Tr
Pineapple & ginger fruit					
spread, 1 tsp	7	1.9	0.1	–	Tr
Raspberry conserve, 1 tsp	13	3.2	–	–	–
Raspberry fruit spread, 1 tsp:					
diet	6	1.5	–	–	–
organic	7	1.7	0.1	–	Tr
Raspberry jam, 1 tsp:	12	3	n/a	–	–
organic	13	3.2	–	–	–
reduced sugar	9	2.3	n/a	–	–
sucrose free	13	3.2	n/a	–	–
Rhubarb & ginger jam,					
reduced sugar, 1 tsp	10	2.5	–	–	Tr
Seville orange fruit spread, 1 tsp					
reduced sugar	6	1.5	–	–	–
organic	7	1.7	0.1	–	Tr

TIP: Even though most jams and marmalades are relatively low in calories per portion, remember that this depends on the quantity you use. Keep to a teaspoonful and spread it thinly.

Jams & Spreads	Cal (kcal)	Carb (g)	Fibre (g)	Pro (g)	Fat (g)
Strawberry fruit spread, 1 tsp	6	1.4	–	–	–
organic	7	1.7	0.1	–	Tr
Strawberry jam, 1 tsp:					
classic	12	3	n/a	–	–
reduced sugar	9	2.3	n/a	–	–
sucrose free	13	3.2	n/a	–	Tr
Wild blackberry jelly,					
reduced sugar, 1 tsp	11	2.7	0.1	–	–
Wild blueberry fruit spread,					
organic, 1 tsp	7	1.8	0.2	–	–
Nut Butters					
Almond butter, 1 tsp	31	0.3	0.4	1.3	2.8
Cashew butter, 1 tsp	32	0.9	0.2	1.2	2.6
Chocolate nut spread, 1 tsp	28	3.1	n/a	0.3	1.7
Hazelnut butter, 1 tsp	34	0.3	0.3	0.8	3.3
Peanut butter, 1 tsp:					
crunchy	30	0.8	0.3	1.2	2.5
smooth	30	0.7	n/a	1.3	2.4
organic	30	0.6	0.3	1.5	2.4
stripy chocolate	31	1.7	0.2	0.7	2.3
Tahini paste, 1 tsp	30	–	n/a	0.9	2.9

TIP: Don't forget about calories. Nut butters may be low in carbohydrates, but they are high in calories when compared to the same quantity of jam.

Jams & Spreads	Cal (kcal)	Carb (g)	Fibre (g)	Pro (g)	Fat (g)
Savoury Spreads and Pastes					
Beef spread, 1 tsp	10	0.1	n/a	0.9	0.7
Cheese spread, 1 tsp:	10	0.4	–	n/a	0.7
reduced fat	9	0.4	–	0.8	0.5
very low fat	6	0.4	0.1	0.9	0.1
See also under: Dairy					
Chicken spread, 1 tsp	11	0.1	n/a	0.7	0.9
Crab spread, 1 tsp	5	0.1	n/a	0.8	0.2
Fish paste, 1 tsp	8	0.2	n/a	0.7	0.5
Guacamole, 1 tsp:					
reduced fat	7	0.4	n/a	n/a	0.6
Hummus, 1 tsp	9	0.6	n/a	0.4	0.6
Liver pâté, 1 tsp:	17	–	n/a	0.6	1.6
low-fat	10	0.2	Tr	0.9	0.6
Meat paste, 1 tsp	4	0.2	–	0.8	0.6
Mushroom pâté, 1 tsp	12	0.4	–	0.4	0.9
Salmon spread, 1 tsp	9	0.2	–	0.7	0.5
Sandwich spread, 1 tsp	11	1.3	–	0.1	0.6

TIP: Diabetic and reduced-sugar jams might seem tempting, but double-check the ingredients. Aspartame – a sugar substitute – has had a bad press in recent years, with some researchers linking it to an increased risk of developing heart disease and certain cancers. And many low-sugar jams contain polyols like maltitol or mannitol, which can have a surprisingly laxative effect.

Jams & Spreads	Cal (kcal)	Carb (g)	Fibre (g)	Pro (g)	Fat (g)
Sandwich spread, *contd*:					
cucumber, 1 tsp	9	1	–	0.1	0.6
Taramasalata, 1 tsp	25	0.2	n/a	0.2	2.6
Toast toppers, 1 tsp:					
chicken & mushroom	3	0.3	–	0.3	0.1
ham & cheese	5	0.4	–	0.4	0.2
Tzatziki, 1 tsp	6	0.2	n/a	0.4	0.5
Yeast extract, half tsp	11	0.9	0.2	1.9	–

TIP: If you hanker after garlic bread, make the Tuscan version, *fettunta*: rub a slice of toasted sourdough bread with a clove of garlic and then drizzle on a little good olive oil.

Meat & Poultry	Cal (kcal)	Carb (g)	Fibre (g)	Pro (g)	Fat (g)
Cooked Meats					
Bacon, 3 rashers, back (50g):					
dry fried	148	–	n/a	12.1	11
grilled	144	–	n/a	11.6	10.8
microwaved	154	–	n/a	12.1	11.7
Bacon, 3 rashers, middle (50g),					
grilled	154	–	n/a	12.4	11.6
Bacon, 3 rashers, streaky (50g):					
fried	168	–	n/a	11.9	13.3
grilled	169	–	n/a	11.9	13.5
Beef, 100g:					
roast rib	300	–	n/a	29.1	20.4
mince, stewed	209	–	–	21.8	13.5
rump steak, lean, grilled	177	–	–	31	5.9
rump steak, lean, fried	183	–	–	30.9	6.6
sausages, see under Sausages					
silverside, lean only, boiled	184	–	n/a	30.4	6.9
stewing steak, stewed	203	–	n/a	29.2	9.6
topside, lean only, roasted	202	–	n/a	36.2	6.3
topside, lean & fat, roasted	244	–	n/a	32.8	12.5
Beef grillsteaks, grilled,					
100g	305	0.5	n/a	22.1	23.9

TIP: Lean beef is low in fat (and saturates), and is a great source of protein, B vitamins and iron.

Meat & Poultry	Cal (kcal)	Carb (g)	Fibre (g)	Pro (g)	Fat (g)
Burgers, each:					
beefburgers (100g) fried	329	0.1	n/a	28.5	23.9
beefburgers (100g) grilled	326	0.1	n/a	26.5	24.4
quarter-pounder (120g)	305	6.1	0.5	17.5	23.4
chicken burger	140	10	0.5	7.5	7.9
vegetable burger	238	27.7	2.3	3.1	12.7
vegetable quarter-pounder	288	33.6	2.5	6.5	14.4
Black pudding, 2 slices, fried	519	29	n/a	18	37.6
Chicken, 100g:					
breast, grilled	148	–	n/a	32	2.2
breast in crumbs, fried	242	14.8	n/a	18	12.7
breast, stir fried	161	–	n/a	29.7	4.6
1 drumstick, roast	185	–	n/a	25.8	9.1
1 leg quarter, roast (175g)	413	–	n/a	36.6	29.6
light & dark meat, roasted	177	–	n/a	27.3	7.5
light meat, roasted	153	–	n/a	30.2	3.6
Duck, 100g:					
crispy, Chinese style	331	0.3	–	27.9	24.2
meat only, roasted	195	–	.	25.3	10.4
meat, fat & skin, roasted	423	–	n/a	20	38.1

TIP: Don't thicken meat juices with flour to make gravy. Put the roasting dish over an oven ring, add a slug of red wine or sherry and cook at a high temperature, stirring all the while. It will be thinner than your normal gravy, but will also have a delicious flavour.

Meat & Poultry	Cal (kcal)	Carb (g)	Fibre (g)	Pro (g)	Fat (g)
Gammon, joint, boiled, 100g	204	–	n/a	23.3	12.3
Gammon, rashers, grilled, 100g	199	–	n/a	27.5	9.9
Goose, roasted, 100g	301	–	n/a	27.5	21.2
Haggis, boiled, 100g	310	19.2	n/a	10.7	21.7
Kidney, lamb, fried, 100g	188	–	n/a	23.7	10.3
Lamb, 100g:					
breast, lean only, roasted	273	–	n/a	26.7	18.5
breast, lean & fat, roasted	359	–	n/a	22.4	29.9
cutlets, lean only, grilled	238	–	n/a	28.5	13.8
cutlets, lean & fat, grilled	367	–	n/a	24.5	29.9
loin chops, lean only, grilled	213	–	n/a	29.2	10.7
loin chops, lean & fat, grilled	305	–	n/a	26.5	22.1
leg, lean only, roasted	203	–	n/a	29.7	9.4
leg, lean & fat, roasted	240	–	–	28.1	14.2
mince, stewed	208	–	n/a	24.4	12.3
stewed	240	–	n/a	26.6	14.8
shoulder, lean only, roasted	218	–	n/a	27.2	12.1
shoulder, lean & fat, roasted	298	–	n/a	24.7	22.1
Liver, calf, fried, 100g	176	Tr	n/a	22.3	9.6
Liver, chicken, fried, 100g	169	Tr	n/a	22.1	8.9

TIP: Instead of using sugary chutneys with Indian food, opt for yoghurt and cucumber raita or marinated raw onion. Mix thinly sliced onion rings with lemon juice, black pepper and salt; leave to marinate for an hour and then transfer the onion to a serving dish.

Meat & Poultry	Cal (kcal)	Carb (g)	Fibre (g)	Pro (g)	Fat (g)
Liver, lamb, fried, 100g	237	Tr	n/a	30.1	12.9
Oxtail, stewed, 100g	243	–	n/a	30.5	13.4
Pheasant, roasted, 100g	220	–	n/a	27.9	12
Pork, 100g:					
belly rashers, grilled	320	–	n/a	27.4	23.4
loin chops, lean, grilled	184	–	n/a	31.6	6.4
leg, lean only, roasted	182	–	–	33	5.5
leg, lean & fat, roasted	215	–	–	30.9	10.2
steaks	198	–	n/a	32.4	7.6
Pork sausages: see Sausages					
Rabbit, meat only, stewed, 100g	114	–	n/a	21.2	3.2
Sausages:					
beef sausages (2), grilled	313	14.7	0.8	15	22
Cumberland sausages (2)	215	9.8	1	9.9	15.2
Frankfurters (2)	369	2.3	Tr	14.1	33.8
Lincolnshire sausages (2)	345	18	1.3	14.6	23.9
pork sausages (2), fried	347	11.2	n/a	15.7	26.9
Saveloy, 100g	296	10.8	n/a	13.8	22.3
Tongue, fat & skin removed, stewed, 100g	289	–	–	18.2	24
Tripe, dressed, 100g	33	–	n/a	7.1	0.5

TIP: Many meat products from deli counters are either high in fat or have had sugar, colourings and/or starchy fillers added.

Meat & Poultry	Cal (kcal)	Carb (g)	Fibre (g)	Pro (g)	Fat (g)
Turkey, 100g:					
breast fillet, grilled	155	–	n/a	35	1.7
dark meat, roasted	177	–	n/a	29.4	6.6
light meat, roasted	153	–	n/a	33.7	2
Veal, escalope, fried, 100g	196	–	–	33.7	6.8
Venison, haunch, meat only,					
roasted, 100g	165	–	n/a	35.6	2.5
White pudding, 100g	450	36.3	n/a	7	31.8
Cold Meats					
Beef, roasted, 50g					
silverside	69	1.2	Tr	9.6	2.9
topside	79	0.2	n/a	12.5	3
Chicken, roasted breast meat,					
50g	76	0.1	Tr	13.5	2.4
Chorizo, 50g	194	2	–	11.5	15.5
Corned beef, 50g	103	0.5	n/a	13	5.5
Garlic sausage, 50g	95	2.9	0.3	7.7	5.8
Ham & pork, chopped, 50g	138	0.7	0.2	7.2	11.8
Ham, 50g:					
canned	82	1	Tr	6	6
honey-roast	70	1.5	–	11	2.2

TIP: Choose back bacon rather than streaky and trim off the fat before cooking. Grill or dry-fry bacon to avoid adding more fat.

Meat & Poultry	Cal (kcal)	Carb (g)	Fibre (g)	Pro (g)	Fat (g)
Ham, *contd*:					
mustard	62	0.9	–	11.5	1.3
on the bone	68	0.4	0.4	10.5	3
beechwood smoked	49	0.5	–	8.5	1.5
Parma	120	0.1	–	12.5	7.5
Wiltshire	101	0.8	0.6	10	6.4
Haslet, 50g	72	9.5	0.4	6.5	1
Kabanos, 50g	120	0.5	0.3	12	7.5
Liver pâté, 50g	174	0.4	n/a	6.3	16.4
reduced fat	96	1.5	Tr	9	6
Liver sausage, 50g	113	3	n/a	6.7	8.4
Luncheon meat, canned, 50g	140	1.8	n/a	6.5	11.9
Pâté, Brussels, 50g	173	2	0.1	6	15.5
Pepperami, hot, 50g	277	1.3	0.6	9.5	26
Pork salami sausage, 50g	268	0.9	0.1	11	24.5
Pork, 50g:					
luncheon meat	134	1.7	–	7	11
oven-baked	92	0.7	0.4	13	4
Salami, 50g:					
Danish	302	0.3	–	7.8	30
German	198	0.5	–	9.5	17.5
Milano	214	1.5	–	11.5	18
Scotch eggs, 100g	241	13.1	–	12	16
Tongue, lunch, 50g	88	0.2	–	9.8	5.2
Turkey, breast, roasted, 50g	58	0.3	–	12.5	0.7

Pasta & Pizza	Cal (kcal)	Carb (g)	Fibre (g)	Pro (g)	Fat (g)
Pasta					
Dried lasagne sheets,					
cooked weight 100g:					
standard	89	18.1	n/a	3.1	0.4
verdi	93	18.3	n/a	3.2	0.4
Dried pasta shapes,					
cooked weight 100g:					
standard	89	18.1	n/a	3.1	0.4
verdi	93	18.3	n/a	3.2	0.4
Fresh egg pasta, 100g:					
conchiglie, penne, fusilli	170	31	1.4	7	2
lasagne sheets	150	29	4.6	6	1.1
spaghetti	129	24	1	5	1.4
tagliatelle	129	24	1	5	1
Macaroni, boiled, 100g	86	18.5	n/a	3	0.5
Spaghetti, cooked weight 100g:					
dried, egg	104	22.2	n/a	3.6	0.7
wholemeal	113	23.2	n/a	4.7	0.9
Stuffed fresh pasta, 100g:					
four cheese tortellini	133	20.1	0.9	5.6	3.3
spinach & ricotta tortellini verdi	163	24	2.7	6	4.5

TIP: If you can't avoid pasta or pizza you can moderate their effects by choosing a healthy sauce such as fresh tomato, or selecting a plain, thin-based pizza and accompanying it with a green salad.

Pasta & Pizza	Cal (kcal)	Carb (g)	Fibre (g)	Pro (g)	Fat (g)
Stuffed fresh pasta, *contd*:					
ham & cheese tortellini	170	13	1.7	6	6
cheese & porcini ravioli	164	21.6	2.8	7.8	5.2
Pasta Sauces					
Amatriciana, fresh, low fat, 100ml	155	5	1	4.4	13
Arrabbiata, fresh, low fat, 100ml	48	7	0.7	1.2	1.7
Bolognese, 100ml	161	2.5	n/a	11.8	11.6
Carbonara:					
fresh, 100ml	196	4.8	0.5	6	17
fresh, low fat, 100ml	81	5	0.5	5	4.5
Pesto:					
fresh, homemade, 100ml	45	6	1.4	2.2	1.3
green pesto, jar, 100ml	374	5	0.8	5	39
red pesto, jar, 100ml	358	3.1	0.4	4.1	36.6
Tomato & basil, fresh, 100ml	51	8.8	1.3	1.8	0.9
Canned Pasta					
Ravioli in tomato sauce, 200g can	146	26.4	0.6	6.2	1.6
Spaghetti bolognese, 200g can	158	26.4	1	6.8	3

TIP: Stuffed pasta has a much higher fat content than plain pasta.

Pasta & Pizza	Cal (kcal)	Carb (g)	Fibre (g)	Pro (g)	Fat (g)
Spaghetti hoops, 200g	106	22.2	1	3.4	0.4
Spaghetti in tomato sauce,					
200g can	122	26	1	3.4	0.4
diet, 200g	100	20.2	1.2	3.6	0.4
Spaghetti with sausages in					
tomato sauce, 200g	176	21.6	1	7	6.8
Spicy pepperoni pasta,					
200g can	166	18.2	1	5.8	7.8
Spicy salsa twists, 200g	150	21.8	1.6	5.4	4.6
Pasta Ready Meals					
Bolognese shells Italiana,					
diet, per 100g	71	9.6	0.8	5.2	1.3
Canneloni bolognese,					
per 100g	149	11.8	n/a	6.1	8.3
Deep pasta bake, chicken &					
tomato, per 100g	95	13	1.3	4.5	3
Lasagne, each	191	14.6	n/a	9.8	10.8
vegetable, per 100g	110	12.6	0.9	5.3	4.7
Pasta bolognese, per 100g	375	54	n/a	18	9.6
Ravioli bianche, 100g	200	29.7	n/a	9.6	4.7

TIP: If you find one brand of wholemeal pasta stodgy, then try another; they have improved a lot recently.

Pasta & Pizza	Cal (kcal)	Carb (g)	Fibre (g)	Pro (g)	Fat (g)
Spaghetti bolognese, per pack	445	60	3.7	26	11
Pizza					
Cheese & onion deep filled pizza, 100g slice	223	30.3	1.3	8.4	8.2
Cheese & tomato pizza, 100g slice:	235	24.8	1.5	9	11.8
deep pan base	249	35.1	n/a	12.4	7.5
French bread base	230	31.4	–	10.6	7.8
thin base	277	33.9	n/a	14.4	10.3
French bread pizza, 100g slice	240	31	1.5	11	7.5
Ham & mushroom pizza, 100g slice	227	29.5	1.1	11.4	7.5
Pepperoni & sausage pizza, 100g slice	303	28.1	2.2	11.6	16
Pepperoni deep crust pizza, 100g slice	263	29.2	1.7	10.6	11.5
Pizza bases, 20cm diameter:					
deep pan	298	56	n/a	8.5	4.4
standard	298	56	n/a	8.5	4.4
stone baked	274	55	n/a	8.5	2.2
Pizza topping, 100g:					
spicy tomato	66	9	1	1.6	2.6
tomato, cheese, onion & herbs	80	8.1	0.9	3	4
tomato, herbs & spices	67	9.4	0.8	1.5	2.6

Rice & Noodles	Cal (kcal)	Carb (g)	Fibre (g)	Pro (g)	Fat (g)
Rice, cooked					
Arborio rice, 75g	105	23.3	0.3	2.2	0.3
Basmati rice, 75g	113	22.4	n/a	2	1.7
Brown rice, 75g	106	24	0.6	2	0.6
Egg fried rice, 75g	156	19.3	0.3	3.2	8
Long grain rice, 75g	103	22.6	–	2.1	0.3
Long grain & wild rice, 75g	104	27.8	–	3.4	0.4
Pilau rice, 75g	106	23	0.5	2.7	0.4
Pudding rice, 75g	107	24.2	0.2	1.9	0.3
Risotto rice, 75g	105	23.3	0.3	2.2	0.3
Short grain rice, 75g	108	26	0.7	2	0.3
White rice:					
plain, 75g	104	23.2	0.1	2	1
easy cook, 75g	104	23.2	n/a	2	1
Wholegrain rice, 75g	102	21.2	0.6	2.7	0.7
Noodles, cooked					
Egg noodles, 75g	47	9.8	0.5	2	0.4
Stir fry noodles, 75g	107	23.8	1.1	2.2	0.4
Thai rice noodles, 75g	108	26	0.7	2	0.3
Thread noodles, 75g	51	7.4	–	1.8	1.5

TIP: You don't just need to watch the quantity of rice you eat; you also need to make sure it is not overcooked. Cooking breaks down the starches, so keep it nutty.

Snacks & Nibbles	Cal (kcal)	Carb (g)	Fibre (g)	Pro (g)	Fat (g)
Crisps					
Cheese corn snacks, per pack (21g)	110	11.3	0.2	1.7	6.3
Hoop snacks, per pack (27g)	175	20.5	0.6	1.1	9.7
Potato crisps:					
cheese & onion, per pack (34.5g)	176	17.9	1.6	2.1	10.7
lightly salted, 25g	121	13.8	1.3	1.6	6.7
mature cheddar with chives, 25g	120	13.6	1.3	2	6.4
pickled onion, per pack (34.5g)	173	17.6	1.6	1.9	10.6
prawn cocktail, per pack (34.5g)	180	16.9	1.5	2	11.6
ready salted, per pack (34.5g)	179	17.8	1.6	1.9	11.1
roast chicken, (light), per pack (28g)	176	17.9	1.7	2.1	10.7
salsa with mesquite, 25g	116	13.8	1.4	1.5	6.1
salt & vinegar, per pack (34.5g)	173	17.7	1.5	1.8	10.6
salt & vinegar, (light), per pack (28g)	112	14.6	1.4	1.8	5

TIP: Don't forget to eat two snacks a day to keep your blood sugar levels steady; just make sure they're good for you. Take batons of carrot, apples and oatcakes to work. If there's nothing healthy to hand, you're more likely to be tempted by crisps or chocolate.

Snacks & Nibbles	Cal (kcal)	Carb (g)	Fibre (g)	Pro (g)	Fat (g)
Potato crisps, *contd:*					
sea salt with balsamic					
vinegar, 25g	122	13.4	1.2	1.7	6.9
smokey bacon, per pack (34.5g)	181	16.9	1.5	2	11.6
Quavers, per pack (20g)	103	12.2	0.2	0.6	5.8
Wheat crunchies:					
bacon flavour, per pack (35g)	172	19.6	1.4	3.4	8.9
salt & vinegar, per pack (35g)	170	19.1	0.9	3.7	8.7
spicy tomato, per pack (35g)	172	19.6	1.4	3.3	8.9
Worcester sauce, per pack (35g)	172	19.7	1.4	3.3	8.9
Nibbles					
Bombay mix, 50g	254	19.2	5.3	5.6	17.2
Breadsticks, each	21	3.6	0.2	0.6	0.4
Japanese rice crackers, 50g	200	39.5	0.3	4.7	2.6
Nachos, 100g	230	31	–	4	10
Olives, 15g black	32	3.4	1.7	0.2	1.0
Peanuts & raisins, 50g	237	15.9	2.4	8.8	15.3
yoghurt coated, 50g	233	27.2	1	4.5	12.9
Popcorn					
candied, 50g	240	38.8	n/a	1.1	10
plain, 50g	297	24.4	n/a	3.1	21.4

TIP: Watch plain popcorn – its calorie count is high.

Snacks & Nibbles	Cal (kcal)	Carb (g)	Fibre (g)	Pro (g)	Fat (g)
Poppadums, each:					
fried in veg oil	92	9.7	–	4.4	4.2
spicy, microwaved	64	10.7	3.2	5	0.1
Prawn crackers, 25g	77	10.3	0.3	0.2	3.9
Tortilla chips					
chilli flavour, 50g	248	31	n/a	3.5	13
cool original, per pack (40g)	204	25	1.4	3	10.5
jalapeño cheese flavour, 50g	260	30.5	n/a	3.5	13.5
pizza, per pack (40g)	202	23	1.4	3	11
salsa flavour, 50g	247	32.5	n/a	3.5	13
salted, 50g	230	30	2.5	3.8	11.3
tangy cheese, per pack (40g)	204	23	1.2	3.2	11
Trail mix, 50g	216	18.6	n/a	4.6	14.3
Twiglets, 50g	192	28.7	5.7	6.2	5.9
curry	225	28	3	4	10.7
tangy	227	28	2.8	4	2.8
Dried Fruit					
Apple rings, 25g	60	15	2.4	0.5	0.1
Apricots, 25g	40	9.1	n/a	1	0.2
Banana, 25g	55	13.4	2.4	0.8	0.2

TIP: Drain some black olives in brine and rinse well under running water; put them in a bowl, add some chopped fresh herbs and a drizzle of olive oil. Stir well and serve.

Snacks & Nibbles	Cal (kcal)	Carb (g)	Fibre (g)	Pro (g)	Fat (g)
Banana chips, 25g	133	16.2	2	0.4	7.4
Currants, 25g	67	17	n/a	0.6	0.1
Dates, flesh & skin, 25g	68	17	n/a	0.8	0.1
Figs, 25g	57	13.2	n/a	0.9	0.4
Fruit salad, 25g	46	11.1	1.8	0.8	0.2
Mixed fruit, 25g	67	17	n/a	0.6	0.1
Pineapple, diced, 25g	87	21	0.9	–	Tr
Prunes, 25g	40	9.6	1.6	0.7	0.1
Raisins, seedless, 25g	72	17.3	0.5	0.5	0.1
Sultanas, 25g	69	17.4	0.5	0.7	0.1
Nuts and Seeds					
Almonds:					
weighed with shells, 50g	115	1.3	1.4	3.9	10.3
flaked/ground, 25g	158	1.8	1.8	6.3	14
Brazils:					
weighed with shells, 50g	157	0.7	1.9	3.3	15.7
kernel only, 25g	170	0.8	1.3	3.5	17
Cashews:					
kernel only, 25g	144	4.5	0.8	4.5	12
pieces, 25g	156	4.3	0.8	6	12.7

TIP: Hummus makes a great dip, and is rich in B vitamins. Make your own, blending cooked chickpeas, some of their cooking liquid, tahini (sesame seed paste), lemon juice, garlic and a little olive oil.

Snacks & Nibbles	Cal (kcal)	Carb (g)	Fibre (g)	Pro (g)	Fat (g)
Chestnuts, kernel only, 25g	43	9.2	n/a	0.5	0.7
Coconut: *see under* Fruit					
Hazelnuts:					
weighed with shell, 50g	124	1.2	1.3	2.7	12.1
kernel only, 25g	167	1.5	1.5	4.3	16
Hickory nuts: *see* Pecans					
Macadamia nuts, salted, 50g	374	2.4	n/a	4	38.8
Mixed nuts, 25g	152	2	n/a	5.7	13.5
Monkey nuts: *see* Peanuts					
Peanuts:					
plain, weighed with shells, 50g	195	4.3	2.2	8.9	15.9
plain, kernel only, 25g	141	3.1	–	6.5	11.5
dry roasted, 50g	295	5.2	n/a	12.9	24.9
roasted & salted, 50g	301	3.6	n/a	12.4	26.5
Pecans, kernel only, 25g	175	1.5	1.2	2.8	17.5
Pine nuts, kernel only, 25g	172	1	n/a	3.5	17.2
Pistachios, weighed with shells, 50g	83	2.3	1.7	2.5	7.7
Poppy seeds, 10g	56	1.9	–	2.1	4.4
Pumpkin seeds, 25g	142	3.8	1.3	6.1	11.4
Sesame seeds, 10g	64	0.6	0.7	2.3	5.8
Sunflower seeds, 25g	145	4.7	1.5	5	11.9

TIP: Consider alternatives to nuts. Pumpkin seeds are rich in minerals and are delicious toasted in a dry frying pan, as are sunflower seeds.

Snacks & Nibbles	Cal (kcal)	Carb (g)	Fibre (g)	Pro (g)	Fat (g)
Walnuts:					
weighed with shell, 50g	148	0.7	0.8	3.2	14.7
halves, 25g	172	0.8	0.9	3.7	17.1
Dips					
Curry & mango dip, 100g	334	6.1	–	4.5	32.4
Mexican dips, 100g:					
guacamole	140	86	n/a	n/a	12.2
Mexican bean	89	12.1	2.4	2.7	3.3
spicy	324	4.8	–	4.7	31.7
Hummus, 100g	187	11.6	n/a	7.6	12.6
Onion & chive dip, 100g	283	5.6	0.5	4.6	26.9
Salsa, 100g					
cheese	143	9.3	n/a	2.5	10.7
cool, organic	141	6.3	1.2	1.1	0.4
Salsa, *contd*:					
hot, organic	141	6.2	1.1	1.1	0.4
picante	28	4.6	–	1.4	0.5
Sour-cream based dips, 100g	360	4	n/a	2.9	37
Taramasalata, 100g	504	4.1	n/a	3.2	52.9
Tzatziki, 100g	66	1.9	n/a	3.8	4.9

TIP: Don't keep nuts too long as the oils they contain will go rancid. Buy little and often.

Soup	Cal (kcal)	Carb (g)	Fibre (g)	Pro (g)	Fat (g)
Canned Soups					
Beef broth, 200ml	86	13.8	2	4.4	1.4
Beef consommé, 200ml	26	1.4	–	5.2	Tr
Beef & vegetable soup, 200ml	96	14.4	2	5.8	1.6
Broccoli soup, 200ml	90	11.8	0.8	2.6	3.6
Broccoli & potato soup, 200ml	62	11.6	1.4	2.6	0.6
Carrot & butter bean soup, 200ml	108	154	3.4	3.2	3.8
Carrot & coriander soup, 200ml	82	12	1.6	1.6	3
Carrot & lentil soup, *low calorie*, 200ml	62	12	1.6	2.8	0.2
Carrot, parsnip & nutmeg organic, 200ml	54	11.4	2	1.4	0.4
Chicken broth, 200ml	68	10.8	1.2	3	0.8
Chicken soup, *low calorie*, 200ml	60	8.2	–	2.4	2
Chicken & ham, 200ml	92	13.8	1.4	4.3	2
low calorie	59	8.8	0.9	1.1	2.2
Chicken & sweetcorn soup, 200ml	78	12.4	1.2	3.2	1.8
Chicken & vegetable soup, 200ml	72	12.2	2.4	3.4	1

TIP: The liquid used for cooking lentils makes an excellent base for a strong-flavoured soup. Reserve it if it's not needed for the lentil dish itself.

Soup	Cal (kcal)	Carb (g)	Fibre (g)	Pro (g)	Fat (g)
Chicken & white wine soup, 200ml	94	7.6	n/a	1.8	6.4
Chicken noodle soup, *low calorie*, 200ml	34	6.2	0.4	1.4	0.2
Cock-a-leekie soup, 200ml	46	8.2	0.6	1.8	0.6
Consommé, 200ml	16	1.2	n/a	3	–
Cream of asparagus, 200ml	134	12	0.4	2.2	8.6
Cream of celery soup, 200ml	92	6	n/a	1.2	7.2
Cream of chicken soup, 200ml	138	12.2	0.2	3.6	8.4
Cream of chicken & mushroom, 200ml	100	9.2	0.2	3.2	5.6
Cream of mushroom, 200ml	126	11	0.2	1.8	8.2
Cream of tomato, 200ml	114	13.2	0.8	1.8	6
Creamy chicken with vegetables, fresh soup, 200ml	194	11	0.8	3.8	15
Cullen skink, 200ml	172	15.4	0.8	12.8	6.6
French onion soup, 200ml	42	8.6	0.8	1.4	0.2
Garden pea & mint fresh soup, 200ml	124	12.2	3	4.6	6.4
Italian bean & pasta soup, 200ml	84	15.8	2.2	4	0.6
Lentil soup, 200ml	80	14.8	2	4.6	0.4

TIP: Don't use potatoes to thicken soup. Choose soups that don't need extra thickening, or use a rough purée of cooked haricot beans.

Soup	Cal (kcal)	Carb (g)	Fibre (g)	Pro (g)	Fat (g)
Lobster bisque, 200ml	92	8.2	0.4	6	4
Mediterranean tomato, 200ml	66	13.6	1.4	2	0.4
Minestrone soup:					
chunky fresh, 200ml	68	11.8	1.8	2.6	1.2
Miso, 200ml	40	4.7	–	2.6	1.2
Mulligatawny beef curry soup					
200ml	94	14.6	1.2	10.4	1.8
Mushroom soup:					
low calorie, 200ml	54	8.8	0.2	2	1.2
Oxtail soup, 200ml	74	13	0.6	3.2	1
Parsnip & carrot:					
low calorie, 200ml	50	10.6	1.8	1	0.4
Pea & ham, 200ml	110	16.6	2.4	6	2.2
Potato & leek, 200ml	90	16.2	1.6	2.2	1.8
Royal game, 200ml	82	12.4	0.4	5.6	1
Scotch broth, 200ml	94	15	1.8	3.8	2
Spicy parsnip, 200ml	102	12.2	3	2.2	5
Spicy tomato & rice with					
sweetcorn, 200ml	90	18.4	1	2.6	0.6
Spring vegetable soup, 200ml	62	12.4	1.4	1.6	0.8

TIP: Croûtons are not the only garnish for soup; try chopped basil over tomato soup or finely chopped cucumber over fennel soup. A few roughly chopped walnuts make a good croûton substitute when you want something crunchier. Slivers of chilli can be added to spicy soups.

Soup	Cal (kcal)	Carb (g)	Fibre (g)	Pro (g)	Fat (g)
Thai chicken with noodles, 200ml	94	13.6	0.6	3.4	0.8
Tomato soup:					
low calorie, 200ml	52	9.4	0.6	1.4	1.0
Vegetable soup, 200ml	86	16.4	1.8	2	1.4
chunky fresh, 200ml	80	15.4	2.2	3.2	0.6
low calorie, 200ml	62	11.8	1.8	2	0.6
Winter vegetable soup, 200ml	92	16.4	2.2	5.6	0.4
low calorie, 200ml	62	12.0	1.6	3.2	0.2
Sachet/Cup Soups					
Beef & tomato cup soup, per sachet	83	15.8	1	1.4	1.6
Broccoli & cauliflower:					
thick & creamy, per sachet	107	13.7	2.7	1.6	5.1
low calorie, per sachet	59	10	0.5	0.9	1.7
Cajun spicy vegetable low calorie soup, per sachet	52	9.4	1.6	1.7	0.8
Cheese & broccoli cup soup, per sachet	160	23.5	1.9	5.2	5

TIP: If soup burns and sticks to the bottom of the pot, decant the unburnt ingredients carefully into a clean pan then check the taste. If it tastes burnt, you won't be able to rescue it and will have to start again. Otherwise, just carry on with the decanted soup.

Soup	Cal (kcal)	Carb (g)	Fibre (g)	Pro (g)	Fat (g)
Chicken soup, cup soup					
per sachet	83	8.3	1.4	1.1	5
Chicken & leek cup soup,					
per sachet	96	12.2	1.7	1.2	4.7
Chicken & mushroom					
per sachet:	132	20.2	1.3	3.7	4
low calorie	60	9	0.9	1.3	2.1
Chicken & sweetcorn soup:					
low calorie, per sachet	55	8.5	0.9	1.2	1.8
Chicken noodle soup:					
per sachet	96	17	0.7	4.3	1.2
Chicken, noodle & vegetable:					
low calorie, per sachet	55	10	1.2	1.6	1
Chinese chicken cup soup					
per sachet	101	19.1	2	3.5	1.2
Cream of asparagus cup soup,					
per sachet	134	18	2.3	0.7	6.6
Cream of chicken & vegetable,					
cup soup, per sachet	137	18	2.2	1.3	6.6
Cream of mushroom, cup soup					
per sachet	121	15.2	2	0.9	6.3

TIP: Be very wary of adding salt to any stock or vegetable cooking water you are going to use for soup, as its flavour becomes intensified. Peppercorns make stock cloudy and impart a rather acrid, burnt taste.

Soup	Cal (kcal)	Carb (g)	Fibre (g)	Pro (g)	Fat (g)
Cream of vegetable cup soup, per sachet	135	17.3	2.8	1.8	6.5
Creamy potato & leek cup soup, per sachet	109	15.5	3	1.9	4.4
Golden vegetable:					
cup soup, per sachet	83	14.3	0.9	1.1	2.4
low calorie, per sachet	58	9.7	1.5	1.1	1.7
Hot & sour cup soup, sachet	91	18.7	1.2	2.5	0.7
Leek & potato low calorie, per sachet	57	10.2	0.5	0.9	1.4
Mediterranean tomato:					
low calorie per sachet	58	9.6	0.7	1.1	1.7
Minestrone soup:					
cup soup, per sachet	98	16.5	1.2	1.6	2.8
low calorie, per sachet	56	9.9	1.3	1.3	1.2
Oxtail soup, per sachet	83	11.2	0.8	2.2	3.3
Spicy vegetable cup soup, per sachet	109	22.3	1.2	2.9	1
Tomato cup soup, per sachet	92	17.2	0.7	0.7	2.3
Tomato & vegetable cup soup, per sachet	108	18.4	2.1	2.8	2.6

Vegetables	Cal (kcal)	Carb (g)	Fibre (g)	Pro (g)	Fat (g)
Artichokes, 1 globe	18	2.7	–	2.8	0.2
Artichoke, Jerusalem, boiled, 90g	37	9.5	–	1.4	0.1
Asparagus, 6 spears, boiled	21	1.1	n/a	2.7	0.6
Aubergine, half medium, fried	151	1.4	n/a	0.6	16
Avocado, half	160	1.6	n/a	1.6	16.4
Bamboo shoots, raw, 75g	5	0.8	0.2	0.5	0.1
Beans, broad, boiled, 75g	61	8.8	n/a	5.9	0.5
Beans, French, 100g boiled	25	4.7	n/a	1.7	0.1
Beans, runner, 50g, trimmed, boiled	9	1.2	n/a	0.6	0.3
Beansprouts, mung, 25g:					
raw	8	1	n/a	0.7	0.1
stirfried in blended oil	18	0.6	n/a	0.5	1.5
Beetroot, 90g:					
pickled	98	23.4	n/a	0.9	0.1
boiled	41	8.6	n/a	2.1	0.1
Broccoli, florets, boiled, 60g	14	0.7	n/a	1.9	0.5
Brussels sprouts, 6 trimmed, boiled	49	4.9	n/a	4.1	1.8

TIP: Cos lettuce keeps well in the fridge, has an excellent flavour and the smaller leaves make efficient and tasty scoops for dips. Always wash the leaves and dry them in a salad spinner or tea towel.

Vegetables	Cal (kcal)	Carb (g)	Fibre (g)	Pro (g)	Fat (g)
Cabbage (Savoy, Summer), 75g:					
trimmed	20	3.1	n/a	1.3	0.3
shredded & boiled	12	1.7	n/a	0.8	0.3
Spring greens, raw	25	2.3	n/a	2.3	0.8
Spring greens, boiled	15	1.2	n/a	1.4	0.5
white	20	3.7	1.6	1.0	0.2
Carrot:					
1 medium, raw	35	7.9	n/a	0.6	0.3
1 medium, raw (young)	34	6.8	n/a	0.8	0.6
grated, 40g	15	3.2	1	0.2	0.1
boiled (frozen), 80g	18	3.8	1.8	0.3	0.2
boiled (young), 80g	18	3.5	n/a	0.5	0.3
Cassava, 100g:					
baked	155	40.1	1.7	0.7	0.2
boiled	130	33.5	1.4	0.5	0.2
Cauliflower, 100g:					
raw	34	3.0	n/a	3.6	0.9
boiled	28	2.1	n/a	2.9	0.9
Celeriac, 100g:					
flesh only, raw	29	5	0.4	1.3	0.4
flesh only, boiled	15	1.9	3.2	0.9	0.5

TIP: Sweet potatoes, the roots of a tropical vine, have a lower GL than true potatoes. Bake them in foil in a medium oven until they are soft. When the foil parcel gives to the touch, they are ready.

Vegetables	Cal (kcal)	Carb (g)	Fibre (g)	Pro (g)	Fat (g)
Celery, 100g:					
stem only, raw	7	0.9	n/a	0.5	0.2
stem only, boiled	8	0.8	n/a	0.5	0.3
Chicory, 100g	11	2.8	n/a	0.5	0.6
Corn-on-the-cob					
boiled, 1 medium cob	76	13.3	n/a	2.9	1.6
mini corncobs, boiled, 100g	24	2.7	2.0	2.5	0.4
See also: Sweetcorn					
Courgettes (zucchini):					
trimmed, 50g	9	0.9	n/a	0.9	0.2
trimmed, boiled, 75g	14	1.5	n/a	1.5	0.3
trimmed, baked, 75g	16	1	n/a	1.1	0.2
fried in corn oil, 75g	47	2	n/a	2	3.6
Cucumber, trimmed, 75g	8	1.1	n/a	0.5	0.1
Eggplant: *see* Aubergine					
Fennel, Florence					
boiled, 75g	8	1.1	n/a	0.7	0.2
Garlic, half tsp purée or					
1 clove, crushed	60	1.8	0.9	0.4	5.7
Gherkins,					
pickled, 75g	11	2	n/a	0.7	0.1
Ginger root, half tsp, grated	–	0.1	–	–	–

TIP: Try not to peel vegetables; removing the peel reduces the fibre content and also removes nutrients just below the skin.

Vegetables	Cal (kcal)	Carb (g)	Fibre (g)	Pro (g)	Fat (g)
Greens, spring: *see* Cabbage					
Gumbo: *see* Okra					
Kale, curly, 40g:					
raw	13	0.6	n/a	1.4	0.6
shredded, boiled	10	0.4	n/a	1	0.4
Kohlrabi, 85g:					
raw	20	3.1	1.9	1.4	0.2
boiled	15	2.6	1.6	1.0	0.2
Ladies' Fingers: *see* Okra					
Leeks:					
trimmed, 60g	13	1.7	n/a	1.0	0.3
chopped, boiled, 100g	21	2.6	n/a	1.2	0.7
Lettuce, 1 cup (30g):					
green	4	0.5	n/a	0.2	0.2
iceberg	4	0.6	n/a	0.2	0.1
mixed leaf	5	0.9	0.8	0.3	–
Mediterranean salad leaves	6	0.9	0.5	0.3	0.1
spinach, rocket & watercress	7.5	0.4	0.4	0.9	0.3
Mange-tout, 50g:					
raw	16	2.1	n/a	1.8	0.1
boiled	13	1.7	n/a	1.6	0.1
stir-fried	36	1.8	n/a	1.9	2.4

TIP: When cooking red cabbage, add a little vinegar to the water to stop it from turning purple.

Vegetables	Cal (kcal)	Carb (g)	Fibre (g)	Pro (g)	Fat (g)
Marrow:					
flesh only, 50g	6	1.1	n/a	0.3	0.1
flesh only, boiled, 75g	7	1.2	n/a	0.3	0.2
Mooli: *see* Radish, white					
Mushrooms, common, 40g:					
raw	5	0.2	n/a	0.7	0.2
boiled	4	0.2	0.4	0.7	0.1
fried in oil	63	0.1	n/a	1	6.5
canned	5	Tr	0.5	0.8	0.2
Mushrooms, oyster, 30g	2	–	0.1	0.5	0.1
Mushrooms, shiitake:					
boiled, 40g	22	4.9	–	0.6	0.1
dried, 20g	59	12.8	–	1.9	0.2
Neeps (Scotland): *see* Swede					
Okra (gumbo, ladies' fingers):					
raw, 25g	10	2	–	0.5	–
boiled, 30g	8	0.8	n/a	0.8	0.3
stir-fried, 30g	81	1.3	n/a	1.3	7.8
Onions:					
raw, flesh only, 30g	11	2.4	n/a	0.4	0.1
boiled, 40g	7	1.5	0.3	0.2	–
cocktail, drained, 40g	6	1.2	n/a	0.2	–

TIP: Toss fresh baby spinach leaves in a little gently warmed olive oil and sprinkle dry-fried pine nuts and chopped almonds over the top.

Vegetables	Cal (kcal)	Carb (g)	Fibre (g)	Pro (g)	Fat (g)
Onions, *contd*:					
fried in vegetable oil, 40g	66	5.6	n/a	0.9	4.5
pickled, drained, 40g	10	2.0	n/a	0.4	0.1
Parsnips, trimmed, peeled,					
boiled, 80g	53	10.3	n/a	1.3	1.0
Peas:					
no pod, 75g	62	8.5	n/a	5.1	1.1
boiled, 90g	71	9.0	n/a	6.0	1.4
canned, 90g	72	12.2	n/a	4.8	0.8
Peas, mushy, canned, 100g	81	13.8	n/a	5.8	0.7
Peas, processed, canned, 100g	99	17.5	n/a	6.9	0.7
See also: Petit pois					
See also under: Beans, Pulses					
and Cereals					
Peppers:					
green, raw, 40g	6	1.0	n/a	0.3	0.1
green, boiled, 50g	9	1.3	n/a	0.5	0.2
red, raw, 40g	13	2.6	n/a	0.4	0.2
red, boiled, 50g	17	3.5	n/a	0.6	0.2
yellow, raw, 40g	10	2.1	0.7	0.5	0.1
chilli, 15g	3	0.1	n/a	0.4	0.1

TIP: Grate celeriac into fine strips, cook it briefly in boiling water then chill it in cold water. Serve with a dressing made from low-fat crème fraîche with a little Dijon mustard mixed in.

Vegetables	Cal (kcal)	Carb (g)	Fibre (g)	Pro (g)	Fat (g)
Peppers, *contd*:					
jalapeños, 15g	3.3	0.5	n/a	0.2	0.1
Petit pois:					
fresh, 75g	75	13.1	3.1	5.2	0.6
frozen, boiled, 100g	49	5.5	n/a	5	0.9
Potatoes, Chips and Fries					
Chips, 150g:					
crinkle cut, frozen, fried	435	50.1	n/a	5.4	25
French fries, retail	420	51	n/a	5	23.3
homemade, fried	284	45.2	n/a	5.9	10.1
microwave chips	332	48.2	n/a	5.4	14.4
oven chips	243	44.7	n/a	4.8	6.3
straight cut, frozen, fried	410	54	n/a	6.2	20.3
Croquettes, fried in oil, 100g	214	21.6	n/a	3.7	13.1
Hash browns, 100g	153	26.8	n/a	2.9	5
Mashed potato, instant, 125g:					
made with semi-skimmed milk	88	18.5	1.3	3	1.5
made with skimmed milk	83	18.5	1.3	3	0.1
made with water	71	16.9	n/a	1.9	0.1
made up with whole milk	95	18.5	1.2	3	1.5
Potato fritters, 100g	145	16.3	1.2	2	8
Potato waffles, 100g	200	30.3	n/a	3.2	8.2

TIP: Blanch raw onion in boiling water if it's too strong for you.

Vegetables	Cal (kcal)	Carb (g)	Fibre (g)	Pro (g)	Fat (g)
Potatoes, new, 100g:					
boiled, peeled	75	17.8	n/a	1.5	0.3
boiled in skins	66	15.4	n/a	1.4	0.3
canned	63	15.1	n/a	1.5	0.1
Potatoes, old, 90g:					
baked, flesh & skin	122	28.5	n/a	3.5	0.2
baked, flesh only	69	16.2	n/a	2.0	0.1
boiled, peeled	65	15.3	n/a	1.6	0.1
mashed with butter & milk	94	14	n/a	1.6	3.9
roast in oil/lard	134	23.3	n/a	2.6	4.0
Pumpkin, flesh only, boiled, 75g	10	1.7	n/a	0.5	0.2
Radicchio, 30g	4	0.5	0.5	0.4	0.1
Radish, red, 6	7	1.1	n/a	0.4	0.1
Radish, white/mooli, 20g	3	0.6	–	0.2	–
Ratatouille, canned, 115g	58	8.1	1.2	1.2	2.3
Salsify:					
flesh only, raw, 40g	11	4.1	1.3	0.5	0.1
flesh only, boiled, 50g	12	4.3	1.8	0.6	0.2
Shallots, 30g	6	1.0	n/a	0.5	0.1
Spinach:					
raw, one cup, 30g	8	0.5	n/a	0.8	0.2
boiled, 90g	17	0.7	n/a	2.0	0.7
frozen, boiled, 90g	19	0.5	n/a	2.8	0.7
Spring onions, bulbs & tops, 30g	7	0.9	n/a	0.6	0.2

Vegetables	Cal (kcal)	Carb (g)	Fibre (g)	Pro (g)	Fat (g)
Sprouts: *see* Brussels Sprouts					
Squash:					
flesh only, 50g	6	1.1	n/a	0.3	0.1
flesh only, boiled, 75g	7	1.2	n/a	0.3	0.2
Swede, flesh only, boiled, 90g	10	2.1	n/a	0.3	0.1
Sweet potato, boiled, 90g	76	18.5	n/a	1.0	0.3
Sweetcorn, kernels, 80g:					
canned, drained, re-heated	98	21.3	n/a	2.3	1.0
canned, no salt, no sugar	62	13.4	2	2.1	–
Tomatoes:					
1 medium	29	4.7	0.6	1.1	0.6
canned, whole, 100g	16	3	n/a	1	0.1
cherry, 6	31	5.3	1.7	1.2	0.5
1 medium, fried in oil	137	7.5	n/a	1.1	11.6
sun-dried, 30g	63	3.3	2	1.3	4.9
paste, 2 tbsp	27	5	n/a	1.7	0.1
passata, 200g	50	9	0.4	2.8	0.2
chopped, canned, 200g	44	7	n/a	2.2	0.8
Turnip, flesh only, boiled, 60g	7	1.2	n/a	0.4	0.1
Water chestnuts, canned, 40g	11	1.9	1	0.7	0.1
Yam, flesh only, boiled, 90g	120	29.7	n/a	1.5	0.3
Zucchini: *see* Courgettes					

TIP: Roast chunks of Mediterranean vegetables in a teaspoon of olive oil at 200°C/gas mark 6 for about 30 minutes, stirring a couple of times.

Vegetarian	Cal (kcal)	Carb (g)	Fibre (g)	Pro (g)	Fat (g)
Baked beans with vegetable sausages, 200g	210	24.4	5.8	12	7.2
Burgers:					
brown rice & tofu burgers, each	184	10.1	3.2	12.2	10.6
carrot, peanut & onion burgers, each	251	23.5	4.0	8.9	13.5
organic vegeburgers, each	238	27.7	2.3	3.1	12.7
savoury burgers, each	162	9.9	2.6	11.1	8.6
soya and black bean burgers, each	158	11.7	4.5	9.5	8.1
spicy bean burgers, each	234	30.9	7.6	7.3	9.9
vegetable burgers, each	179	20.8	1.7	2.3	9.6
Cauliflower cheese, 100g	365	22	–	18	23
Cheese, vegetarian:					
Double Gloucester, 25g	101	–	–	6.2	8.5
mild Cheddar, 25g	103	–	–	6.4	8.6
Red Leicester, 25g	100	–	–	8.1	8.4
Cornish pasty, each	452	37.3	2.0	11	28.9
Falafel, 4 (100g)	220	23.3	7.6	8	10.5

TIP: Marinate chunks of plain and smoked tofu, onion, peppers, tomatoes and button mushrooms in a teaspoon each of soy sauce (shoyu) and wine vinegar, plus a little Dijon mustard. Thread the tofu and vegetables on skewers, brush lightly with oil and barbecue or grill.

Vegetarian	Cal (kcal)	Carb (g)	Fibre (g)	Pro (g)	Fat (g)
Hummus, 2 tbsp	53	3.3	n/a	2.2	3.6
Lentils, 115g:					
green/brown, boiled	121	19.4	n/a	10.1	0.8
red, split, boiled	115	20.1	n/a	8.7	0.5
Macaroni cheese, individual	470	67	2.4	17	15
Nut roast, 100g:					
courgette & spiced tomato	208	12.5	4.9	11.7	12.3
leek, cheese & mushroom	240	13.2	4.1	13.2	14.9
Onions & garlic sauce, 100g	37	7.7	0.9	1.4	0.1
Pâté, 50g:					
chickpea & black olive	90	7.8	2.2	3.1	5.2
herb	83	3.0	–	3.5	8
herb & garlic	109	3.5	n/a	3.5	9
mushroom	107	3	n/a	3.5	9
red & green pepper	111	4.5	–	3	9
spinach, cheese & almond	86	3.2	1.2	3.6	6.6
Polenta, ready-made, 100g	72	15.7	n/a	1.6	0.3
Quorn, myco-protein, 100g	92	1.9	–	14.1	3.2
Ravioli in tomato sauce, (meatfree), 200g	146	26.4	0.6	6.2	1.6

TIP: Choose soya milk rather than rice milk, but avoid flavoured ones – they are high in calories. Sweetened soya milk is also significantly higher in calories than the unsweetened version.

Vegetarian	Cal (kcal)	Carb (g)	Fibre (g)	Pro (g)	Fat (g)
Red kidney beans:					
small can (200g)	182	27	12.8	16.2	1
boiled, 115g	118	20	n/a	9.7	0.6
Rice drink, 240ml:					
calcium enriched	120	23	–	0.2	2.9
vanilla	118	22.8	–	0.2	2.9
Roast vegetable & tomato					
pasta, 97% fat-free, each	300	56	–	10	3.7
'Sausage' rolls, 100g	273	28.2	2.5	9.7	13.5
'Sausages', 100g (2 sausages)	252	8.6	1.2	23.2	13.8
spicy Moroccan	147	12.7	4.0	9.1	8.4
tomato & basil	147	9.3	3.2	8.6	9.8
Soya bean curd: *see* Tofu					
Soya chunks:					
flavoured, 100g	345	35	4	50	1
unflavoured, 100g	345	35	4	50	1
Soya curd: *see* Tofu					
Soya flour:					
full fat, 100g	447	23.5	n/a	36.8	23.5
low fat, 100g	352	28.2	n/a	45.3	7.2
Soya milk:					
banana flavour, 240ml	180	25.2	2.9	8.6	5

TIP: Many vegetarian ready meals and processed foods are high in trans fats; watch out for hydrogenated fat in the list of ingredients.

Vegetarian	Cal (kcal)	Carb (g)	Fibre (g)	Pro (g)	Fat (g)
Soya milk, *contd*:					
chocolate flavour, 240ml	194	25.7	2.9	9.1	5.8
strawberry flavour, 240ml	154	18.5	2.9	8.6	5
sweetened, 240ml	103	6	Tr	7.4	5.8
unsweetened, 240ml	62	1.2	1.2	5.8	3.8
Soya mince:					
flavoured, 100g	345	35	4	50	1
unflavoured, 100g	345	35	4	50	1
Spaghetti 'bolognese', (meatfree) 200g	172	26.2	1.4	6.2	4.8
Sweet pepper sauce, 100g	89	4.3	0.5	1.5	7.2
Tofu (soya bean curd), 100g:					
smoked	148	1.0	0.3	16	8.9
steamed	73	0.7	n/a	81	4.2
steamed, fried	261	2	n/a	23.5	17.7
tangy, marinated	70	2.0	0.4	7.9	3.4
Vegetable biryani, each	690	74	–	12	38
Vegetable granulated stock, 30g	60	12	0.3	2.6	0.2
Vegetable gravy granules, 50g	155	29.7	1.6	4.2	2.1
Vegetable sauce, 100ml	59	7	2.5	2	2.6
Vegetable stock cubes, each	45	1.4	Tr	1.4	4.1

TIP: A dairy-free smoothie can be made by blending tofu with strawberries and a teaspoonful of honey. Whizz until smooth and drink immediately.

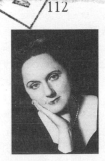

Elizabeth Taylor

Elizabeth Taylor, who was born in Reading, Berkshire, in 1912 and educated at the Abbey School, Reading, worked as a governess and librarian before her marriage in 1936: 'I learnt so much from these jobs,' she wrote, 'and have never regretted the time I spent at them.' She lived in Penn, Buckinghamshire, for almost all her married life. Her first novel, *At Mrs Lippincote's*, appeared in 1945 and was followed by eleven more, together with short stories which were published in various periodicals and collected in five volumes, and a children's book, *Mossy Trotter*. Taylor's shrewd but affectionate portrayals of middle- and upper-middle-class English life soon won her a discriminating audience, as well as staunch friends in the world of letters. Rosamond Lehmann called her 'sophisticated, sensitive and brilliantly amusing, with a kind of stripped, piercing feminine wit'. Elizabeth Taylor died in 1975.

Novels by Elizabeth Taylor

At Mrs Lippincote's
Palladian
A View of the Harbour
A Wreath of Roses
A Game of Hide-and-Seek
The Sleeping Beauty
Angel
In a Summer Season
The Soul of Kindness
The Wedding Group
Mrs Palfrey at the Claremont
Blaming

Short Story Collections

Hester Lilly and Other Stories
The Blush and Other Stories
A Dedicated Man and Other Stories
The Devastating Boys
Dangerous Calm

IN A SUMMER SEASON

Elizabeth Taylor

Introduced by Elizabeth Russell Taylor

virago

TO
JOHN

VIRAGO

Published by Virago Press Limited 1983
Reprinted 1983, 1985, 1988, 1991, 2000, 2006, 2007, 2008,
2010 (twice), 2011, 2012 (three times)

First published in Great Britain by Peter Davies Ltd 1961

A CIP catalogue record for this book
is available from the British Library.

ISBN 978-1-84408-320-6

Printed and bound in Great Britain by
Clays Ltd, St Ives plc

Papers used by Virago are from well-managed forests
and other responsible sources.

MIX
Paper from
responsible sources
FSC® C104740

Virago Press
An imprint of
Little, Brown Book Group
100 Victoria Embankment
London EC4Y 0DY

An Hachette UK Company
www.hachette.co.uk

www.virago.co.uk

Introduction

'She is a young woman who looks as if she never had to wash her gloves!' Ivy Compton-Burnett's estimation was intended to compliment Elizabeth Taylor. Inadvertently, however, it rather played into the hands of early, less discerning critics who regarded her and her work as no more than middle-class conformist. But Ivy Compton-Burnett understood with Proust that 'even if a literary work concerns unintellectual subjects it is nonetheless a product of the intellect'.

The limitations imposed by domestic life on the stockbroker belt in no way deterred Elizabeth Taylor from friendships further afield, with writers whose work was judged 'literary' and not, as was hers, 'occupying a position somewhere between literature and popular fiction'. Ivy Compton-Burnett, Angus Wilson, Elizabeth Bowen and James Agate were among those who recognized her wit, clarity and stylishness and regarded less sympathetic readings of her work as misunderstanding of its subtlety. Her canvas may be small – as is Jane Austen's, with whose work hers has been compared – but she is an incomparable colourist.

Taylor was reticent about disclosing details of her private life, and modest as to her achievements. The fact that she had been a member of the Communist Party in the thirties and throughout her life atheist and a Labour voter shows how skilful she was in creating a credible heroine with whom she sympathized and yet who fell far short of her own intellectual and creative aspirations.

In his book *Elizabeth & Ivy*, Robert Liddell published letters that reveal Taylor as an intelligent, compassionate woman with an acute ear for dialogue and eye for detail, and an unusually retentive memory, faculties that could lead her, she admitted, to lose sight of the wood for the trees. In this novel, details fasten tenaciously to memory. Who could forget the 'little gusts of song' shaken from the housekeeper, or the maiden aunt (who regards breakfast as 'a test of character') bending by a closed door 'not listening . . . but ascertaining'? And who will ever think of bell-ringing without recalling it as an excellent cure for chilblains? What woman victimized by the affectations of her own hairdresser will not remember Elbaire when her practitioner 'with the solemnity of a votary' holds a mirror to the back of her head?

In a Summer Season is Taylor's eighth novel, an entertainment in which the plot – more a storyline – is nugatory. There is no concern with consciousness or big themes. Taylor is on record as saying she could never write about tragedies. There is right and wrong but no good and evil. The novel proceeds in a series of scenes 'rather than in narrative which I find boring', she explained.

Published on the cusp of 'you-never-had-it-so-good' and the Swinging Sixties, the book ignores the events of the decade altogether. Suez, the Wolfenden Commission, the abolition of the death penalty and the power of CND do not detain Taylor. Her canvas is the unsettling heat of early summer in a village in the Thames valley. Nor does she try her hand at working-class realism, becoming fashionable elsewhere. She restricts herself to the portrait of a middle-aged, middle-class housewife living in a comfortable house set in a well-maintained garden presided over by a housekeeper and a gardener.

The temptation is to conflate author and heroine, for their environments are similar and from what the author owned were her preferences – an appreciation of the dailiness of domestic life in ordered countryside, where nothing of a sensational nature is likely to occur – she and Kate share a disposition. The significant difference is that whereas the author had a creative life, her heroine had none. In her personal life Taylor achieved a balance she denied her heroine. The cause for which Kate's suffragist aunt valiantly endured the rigours of Holloway did not ignite the Thames Valley; Kate has no job, nor does she pursue an interest; she cannot develop. Her life is as circular as the novel it defines.

Kate Heron, a widow of means, marries a charmer as attractive to men as to women, the old as to the young. Dermot is ten years younger than Kate and lacks all purpose. He has none of the cultural interests Alan, Kate's late husband aroused in her – Henry James, Beethoven quartets, long country walks – just lust. It is the experience of intense sexual feeling that encourages Kate to overlook Dermot's ignorance and share with him his preferences for darts, drink and race-meetings, not to mention 'kissing in public'. But Kate belongs in time and place to an order of women whose sense of identity is forged by their husbands and her present situation discomposes her. Through Alan she discovered herself, and that identity persists, even if currently starved of nourishment. Once Dermot has been disposed of she will marry Alan's childhood friend, Charles, a man with a job and a house. She will have been returned to old certainties.

In a Summer Season is seen through Kate Heron's eyes. A year past this conventional woman relinquished the world in which husbands support their wives financially for a man who does not conform to that pattern. Hardly surprising that the virus of speculation runs riot through the village, let alone the family. Everyone wonders upon what such a liaison can be founded and for how long it can endure. Lou, Kate's sixteen-year-old daughter, believes her mother is in competition with her twenty-two-year-old son's girlfriends: 'I think my mother gets jealous, and that's why she married Dermot; perhaps she thought that she would be getting someone quite young; who would be a bit like a son, but who would have to take her everywhere with him.'

Aunt Ethel gives the marriage 'five years at most'. She regards Dermot as a parasite, bought with Alan's legacy: 'When the sex goes Kate will think him no bargain.' Mrs Meacock, the housekeeper, reflecting on her own life, observes that whereas she has achieved peace of mind, her employer has traded tranquillity for sex. *In a Summer Season* records the tension between domestic routine and the erotic. Most of the characters are 'blighted' by sex: the whole novel is suffused with the sense that beneath urgent physical pleasure lies permanent unrest. Stability is what is prized in the Thames Valley; Dermot is an erotic diversion from that bourgeois compass reading and can only lead to a dead end.

Kate and Dermot believe they love one another and intermittently they hold dear. But their regard is deflected by self-interest. Taylor is always commended for her ability to convey self-deception. She does so keenly in this book. It is taken for granted in the village that Dermot married Kate for money. But to insist on that judgement as being the only explanation for his driving force is to ignore his unconscious motives.

Dermot is a child who discovers in Kate a mother who desires him, who is more amenable, more pliant than the getting-and-shopping example assigned him by birth. Edwina set him a thoroughly bad example to follow in the first place and, in the second, fell short of gratifying his demands. Kate, well equipped to answer the requirements of a child, treats her husband as such, not only from her deep pockets but also from the deep concern she feels for his future. Kate cannot face the implication of what she is doing by extending her gift for mothering to a husband able to satisfy her lust but unable to interest her, let alone fulfil her. Added to which she is ambivalent in her feelings towards the young; she is both envious and disapproving of them. This places her in an uncomfortable position while she considers whether she should be 'making herself young for her husband'.

Aunt Ethel writes to her friend: 'Take away the physical side and what have you there but disillusion!' The message of Kate and Dermot's experience may lack enchantment but its telling is captivating. Taylor's 'despairing struggle' with her craft results in nice descriptions of place, subtle observations of behaviour and tender reflections on the torments of the affections. But the lasting reward of *In a Summer Season* is the accurate account of a particular type of adult woman in the 1950s, living in the Home Counties. A woman *chosen* by a man for his mate, to bear and rear his children and run his home, exclusively. Kate is so dominated by these twin roles that without one or the other she is disorientated and, being off-balance, plunges into an aberrant relationship. She is, therefore, something of a victim. She continues to lead the morally good life by demonstrating a sense of duty towards her dependent relations, but she leads life at the expense of her own development. She has no access to her deepest needs and appears unaware of having potentialities to fulfil. Whereas the author recognized both obligations to her own life, her heroine sensed conflict between self-fulfilment and the requirements of the common good. This is a conflict that can only be resolved through self-knowledge, the very quality Elizabeth Taylor has created her protagonists to lack.

Elisabeth Russell Taylor
London 1999

At the Beginning of Summer

'AFTER all, I am not a young girl to be intimidated by her,' Kate decided, as she waited outside her mother-in-law's house. When she had reached the stage of thinking that if there were any intimidating to be done she might even do it herself, one of Edwina's foreign girls opened the door.

The house was in a terrace, leading off from a tree-filled London square, and Kate was always surprised to find how much quieter it was than the country. She followed the girl upstairs to the drawing-room. Facing her, as she turned the stairs, was a *trompe-l'œil* panel, designed to lengthen the passage into an endless arcade with recurring statues of Roman emperors set on a black and white chessboard pavement. 'Only it doesn't trompe *my* œil,' she thought.

The drawing-room was all white, except for a sofa and one or two chairs covered in silvery-green silk, and some leaves of the same green arranged amongst white flowers.

Waiting for Edwina, who was probably not up yet, Kate found nothing to look at, nothing interesting left lying about. The room was like a room in an exhibition and she could not imagine any of the beautiful flowers fading or dropping their petals.

Such silence everywhere. The two foreign girls and any kitchen noises they might be obliged to make were two floors down. Overhead, floorboards very softly creaked. 'I have caught her on the hop,' thought Kate. She had always guessed that Edwina lay in bed till noon. How otherwise get through the triviality of the day? She went to one of the windows to see if there were any signs of life in the street below. A milkman in a white coat was defacing the elegance of doorways with groups of pint bottles; at one door,

9

just half a pint—a sad sight, Kate thought, imagining a solitary old lady and a cat.

'Darling,' said Edwina. 'I was just doing my nails and they wouldn't dry.'

She kissed Kate's cheek and held her hands out of harm's way as she did so. Charm bracelets and twisted gold chains slid down from her plump wrists.

'That's a nice suit,' she said in a surprised voice.

Kate had felt just right, perfectly dressed for a day in London, until Edwina had come downstairs. She still thought she could not have chosen better and wondered if what was wrong with the effect—and something was now seen to be—was herself. She was out of doors too much in the country. She hadn't a London face like her mother-in-law's, her skin was a different colour and she looked too healthy for the dark suit—a country woman dressed up in London clothes.

'I don't know how you keep so slim,' Edwina said.

Kate looked complacent, but she knew that if Edwina ever lost her plumpness she would not be half so happy, would be less busy than ever without her Turkish baths and massaging and all the other slimming tricks as they came along and the books she read about it and the articles in magazines, to say nothing of the conversations with her friends.

'And how's that darling son of mine?' Edwina asked but, without waiting for Kate's answer, went out to the landing and began calling down the stairs, 'Paulette, Solange,' then muttered irritably and, shrilling more than ever, called again.

A voice like machine-gun fire began a rattling volley down below and at once, without replying, Edwina came in and slammed the door.

'What do I want indeed! Do they expect me to have long conversations with them hanging over the banisters?'

'Dermot is very well,' said Kate, answering the other question. 'He sent his love of course.'

'He never comes to see me.'

Kate thought, 'Because when he *does* come, you say "Hullo, stranger". No wonder he puts it off.' Trying to avoid a breach for which she knew she would be blamed, she had to come herself, from time to time, and very heavily she always dreaded it.

Paulette or Solange could now be heard dragging herself up the second flight of stairs. At last she stood in the doorway, breathless and sulky.

'Ah, Paulette,' said Edwina, in a light and kindly voice. 'Will you bring up the decanter of whisky from the dining-room, and some ice. A nice lot of ice. You will have whisky, Kate? No? Oh dear. You'll find something else down there, I expect, Paulette. There should be some gin, or some sherry. Forage round. Is sherry all right, Kate? Yes, I'm sure there is some. You understand "sherry", Paulette?' she asked, raising her voice.

'Yes, madame.'

'Whisky, ice, sherry,' Edwina said, ticking off each on her fingers and enunciating carefully, as to an imbecile.

When the girl had gone she sighed.

'It's about Dermot that I want to talk to you,' she told Kate. 'But that we can do over lunch.' She liked to keep people needlessly in suspense, and at the back of her mind Kate now had a feeling of unease. She wondered if her mother-in-law had another of her schemes for Dermot's future and, although she could not guess what it was, her thoughts from then on were busy planning a counter-attack. A look of animation on her face was supposed to hide the fact that she was no longer listening to anything Edwina said. In fact, an admiring or sympathetic murmur from time to time was all that Edwina required, once she was settled passionately to her shopping-talk. Triumphant forays, dignified rebukes (by herself) she described; goods returned and goods tracked down; from the jersey with the pulled thread she drifted to the matched saucer, some trouble with the dry-cleaners, praise from her dressmaker for being long-waisted. (A proper Harrods woman, Dermot, her son, called her.) And all the time Kate was wondering what she could be going to suggest this time and what she herself could say in reply.

Although everything was grand at luncheon, Edwina fussed as if it were all being done for the first time. It was surprising that she, to whom social occasions meant so much, should never have been able to master the art of being a hostess. At meal-times, even with just the family, she became as uncertain as a young bride, quite obviously checked the table to see if all was there that should be, bothered the maid, lost the thread of conversation, became absent-minded when dishes were brought in and stared anxiously and silently as Kate helped herself to some chicken fricassee.

'About Dermot,' she began, when at last Paulette had left the room; then 'Oh', she said repressively, as the girl returned with something she had forgotten. Edwina watched her and saw her out of the room in silence. 'About Dermot,' she said again. Kate was ready. When she chose to speak her voice would be cool, but she did not intend to use it yet.

'I know he's made a good many false starts and had some bad advice,' her mother-in-law went on. 'I'm not blaming you, naturally.'

It would have been wonderful, Kate thought, if she could have found the effrontery to do so, since she had had so long to set him on the right path, and Kate had only had a year.

'He hasn't any plans yet, I suppose?' Edwina asked.

'He is trying to grow mushrooms in one of the outhouses and may make a name for himself that way,' Kate said, and her voice sounded just as she wished it to, light and amused. 'This is very good fricassee, Edwina,' she added.

'Growing mushrooms! I have never heard such nonsense. It isn't fair to you to be so irresponsible and it certainly isn't fair to himself. I hope you are not encouraging him, Kate. It will be the ruin of him if you do. He is grown-up and a married man.'

As this was already known to Kate, she made no reply.

'It was his father's fault for leaving him that bit of money—little as it is, it has sapped his ambition. I can't imagine what all your friends and neighbours say.'

Kate thought it surprising that Edwina could have brought herself to say this. She was afraid that she was blushing now and that her silence appeared stubborn, not off-hand any longer. She drank some water and felt that Edwina was watching it going down her throat.

'You mustn't think I am interfering,' said Edwina, sensing Kate's angry embarrassment. 'But I have been worried lately. I hoped that marriage would make him settle down. Gordon always said it would.' Gordon was her elder son; a model husband and father, too. An actuary. 'Whatever the hell that may be,' Dermot had said.

'His father was the most industrious, the most utterly selfless man,' Edwina went on. 'I can see him now, the minute dinner was over, going off with his papers to his study. He would sit there till midnight. Just as Gordon often does. I have always wondered why Dermot is so different.'

'Perhaps he takes after you,' Kate said. Her voice was bold, and no longer under control.

To her surprise, Edwina's face softened. She looked dreamy and pleased with herself. 'I was certainly rather a handful when I was a girl,' she said. 'Gracious, the escapades, the parties, the young men. "She is like a butterfly and no one will ever manage to catch her," they used to say.'

'Then Patrick caught you and shut you up all alone in the drawing-room, while he went off to work on his papers.'

'It was the beauty of his voice I couldn't escape. The Irish in it. Gordon never had a trace of it and Dermot only when he was trying to get round me. Oh, it was a very happy marriage. I had everything I wanted. He worshipped the ground I walked on. I was just a little bored sometimes in the evenings.'

'Harrods being closed,' thought Kate.

Then the dreamy self-indulgent look suddenly faded and Edwina said briskly: 'Well, I was discussing Dermot with my old friend, Lord Auden. He had always thought a great deal of Dermot, you know.'

'Yes, I thought he was quite in love with him, that time we met.'

'He always asks after him. The other day he was telling me his plans for starting a rather amusing little business—selling Victoriana . . . well, buying it first, I suppose . . . you know those shell flower-arrangements under glass domes and wax fruit and funny old Jubilee mugs. He's been looking for premises. Yesterday I went with him to a place quite near Harrods, but unfortunately there was another shop near by selling the same sort of things.'

'And where does Dermot come in?' It had gone on long enough, Kate decided.

'Lord Auden—Wilfred—wants someone to go into partnership with him and we thought it seems the very thing for Dermot.'

'Victoriana? You amaze me, Edwina. He would break all the glass domes. You can't be serious.'

'It would be much better than doing nothing at all,' Edwina said primly.

'What on earth would he do—dust the shells and wrap up parcels? And how much would Lord Auden pay him for that? Not much, I'll be bound.'

'Wilfred wouldn't pay him anything if they were in partnership.'

'He'd have to put money *into* it?'

But the money would not be Dermot's. It would be Kate's— that left to her by her first husband. The matter was a little delicate and Edwina hesitated.

'Wilfred is sure that it will prove to be a gold-mine,' she said. 'He has the right contacts and such a flair. He has only to start something and everyone follows suit. Moreover, although I am his mother, I think Dermot is very good-looking and has a pleasant personality.'

'And although I am his wife, I agree with you.'

What a complicated little dish those two had been cooking, she thought. Lord Auden, the pink-faced, mincing creature, would get the money he needed and Dermot thrown in—Dermot amongst all the Victoriana; and Edwina would be able to hold her head up again, if her son were no longer living idle on an older woman's money. (He had married her for it, everyone at the Bridge Club must have said behind her back.) He would have to go to London every day, Kate supposed, and his mother could pop into the shop—if such a plain name might be used for it—every day to see him.

She put on a thoughtful expression, as if she were considering the matter with great care while she was eating, but she was really picturing Dermot standing there, hemmed in by rosewood work-tables and whatnots, looking wild and enraged and mystified.

'Of course I . . . we shall have to think it over,' she said.

'But, of *course*, my dear. And then you must meet Wilfred. I'm sure his enthusiasm will infect you.'

Kate had at least another hour with Edwina before she could leave to go to the hairdresser's, and it would be uncomfortable to spend it quarrelling. They talked of other things and Edwina thought that, having sown the seed, she would be clever to let it grow in peace.

So she was all the more astonished when Kate got up to go and, smoothing her gloves, said, 'Well, I have thought it over now, Edwina dear. It is kind of you to be so busy for our sakes, but I must ask you not to let it happen again. Dermot and I like to make our own plans, you see.' Then she put her cheek against Edwina's, smiled and said thank you for her luncheon and was gone.

.   .   .   .   .

In the looking-glass at the hairdresser's, Kate glared at her face as if it were Edwina's. The bearded young man behind her, sensing restlessness, suggested a coloured rinse. 'Rinse' sounded more non-chalant than 'dye'. Kate seemed to him today to be wounded and on the defensive, a mood that came and went, he knew, with women in their forties. She had probably been shopping and found that she needed a larger size in skirts. He was inclined to be a little knowing about women, as he had to be most things to them at one time or another. He switched on different sides of his nature in just as long as it took him to cross the salon from one client to another, and knew when to be sympathetic, reverent, rallying or flirtatious. With Kate he expected a restful interlude. She would ask a few kind questions about his wife and baby and his mother, whose arthritis worried him; then she would pick up a magazine and turn its pages peacefully. He had some clients who watched every hairpin going in, as if they were doubtful of his ability, and others who brought photographs of models and asked to be made to look the same. Kate, from her confidence in him, or her lack of interest, left herself in his hands.

At first, he took up some of her hair and seemed to weigh it, was non-committal as he examined it. 'How has it kept?' he asked.

'Oh, so-so. I found some white hairs in the front.'

He had found them himself some time ago and there were more at the back where she could not see them. White hairs might, of course, account for her mood.

'A rinse would give a more uniform colour,' he said, 'and bring out the copper highlights.'

'How much does it cost?' she asked, without lowering her voice. His salon personality was scandalised, but the self that was buried all day, that came back to life as he made his way home to Harrow by tube in the rush-hour, who was called 'Bert', not 'Elbaire', respected this naked common sense and, meeting her eyes in the mirror, said candidly, 'Twelve-and-six.'

'Very well,' said Kate.

'Amanda, get Madame washed,' he called, turning away. 'He is a nice lad,' thought Kate. Not so very much older than her own son, yet hard-working and responsible—a husband, a father, and such a good boy to his mother, too.

She leant back, as Amanda, who was really Madge, washed her hair, and gradually the different atmosphere soothed her. They were nice young people, busy and comforting, although they had troubles of their own. Love-trouble Amanda had week after week, and Elbaire's baby was teething and kept them awake at nights; yet all they seemed concerned with was making her feel more pleased with herself, brightening her up, bringing out copper highlights that never had been there.

As Elbaire set her hair, she became a little nervous about these highlights and wondered if her twelve-and-sixpence had not been ill-advisedly spent. She had made up her mind when she married Dermot that having a husband ten years younger than herself set a great many booby traps before her—mutton dressed up like lamb being one of them.

Amanda handed the pins and rollers to Elbaire swiftly and efficiently, as if he were a great surgeon to whom she was used to ministering. Although his attention seemed exclusively Kate's, it could not have been, for, from time to time, the girl was sent off on errands to other parts of the salon—to 'take the Countess out' or 'turn Lady Jameson down' or 'see if Mrs Digby-Wetherell needs another five minutes'.

Kate's anger was dwindling, but she still had to plan some sort of account for Dermot of her luncheon with his mother, and to discuss Edwina at all with him put a constraint upon her. Although Dermot would have entirely avoided his mother's company if he could, he was quickly suspicious of any hint of criticism or amusement when other people spoke of her. Lord Auden they could safely laugh about, Kate decided, but she realised that, no matter what she said, ahead of her lay Dermot's touchiness and hurt pride.

She met Elbaire's eyes in the looking-glass, as he put his hands to her temples, lifting the hair a fraction of an inch, so that she would not dare to put her hat on and flatten it. He did not see *her*: his intent gaze was rather that of a portrait-painter, ruthlessly self-absorbed. He looked almost exhausted, as if his confidence in himself had been strained to its limits and, now that his creation was finished, he seemed much too tired to enjoy his triumph. Kate felt she had been taken from the oven and dished up and garnished. Rather more *bouffant* than usual he had made her, he explained— to help out with her high forehead; as for the rinse, although Kate could see no difference, he assured her that it had had its effect. He dropped his hands, looked at her at last.

'Thank you,' he said and smiled and became the nice lad from Harrow again, and then was quickly off across the salon to talk about horse-racing with Mrs Digby-Wetherell.

'You don't like moons, do you, Lady Jameson?' the manicurist shouted to her client under the drier.

A light breeze outside played havoc with her newly *bouffant* hair, as Kate stood at the edge of the pavement waiting for a taxi. She carried her hat.

'I like the hair-style,' said the driver, when at last she found an empty cab. As they drove down Bond Street, he slid the glass partition along and leaned back to shout over his shoulder.

'I always take an interest in the different styles. My daughter's just started as a hairdresser.'

Kate, smoothing her velvet hat, made the expected inquiries. The girl was only a year older than her own daughter, who always seemed babyish compared with the Amandas and Daphnes who, as smart as paint, were out earning their own livings. Louisa, still at school, never used make-up, lived in old jerseys and jeans and had not the faintest idea of anything she could do as a career. Some of this she confided to the taxi-driver. 'You don't look old enough to have a girl of sixteen,' he said.

'I have a son of twenty-two as well.'

His incredulity was lost as the traffic suddenly shot forward, but at the next standstill he leaned back again and said, 'I hope she knows the facts of life—your daughter, I mean. It's a dangerous world for an ignorant young girl. Anyone who drives a cab will tell you that. Though some of them, I must say, know too much. If their mothers guessed what went on, their heads would turn grey. None of that old-fashioned drive twice round the park and hope to hold her hand on the second circuit. Nowadays girls lose their virginity between Claridges and the Ritz and very glad to do so, from all I gather. So-called debs etcetera.'

All the way to the station he gave advice and descriptions of

18

teenage scandals. People were infatuated with adolescence, Kate thought, as if it were the most wonderful thing that ever happened. As a person much confided in, she had learnt how to let her mind wander a little on a tether, and now she looked out of the taxi at the sun flashing high on buildings and thought what a lovely late afternoon it was. The trees in Portman Square were hazy with buds and the sky was as pale as pearls. It was the first spring-like day there had been; behind were months of icy winds, little bouts of snow, thawings, then freezings, a wretched time ever since Christmas.

When she got out of the cab at Marylebone Station, it seemed quite awkward to have to tip the man, they were so much like old friends. The train was in and she bought an evening newspaper and found a corner seat. She glanced at one or two of the woeful head-lines and then leaned back and closed her eyes. They were at Denham before she opened them again.

'Mrs Heron!'

The young girl sitting opposite smiled at her. Who was it, Kate wondered—a Jane, or a Prue, or a Penelope? It was too much to be asked to keep up with them. This one was very pretty—but so were most of them—and just as eager as the others were to be nice to Kate, because of Tom, her son.

She had always tried to be especially kind to Tom's succession of girls and more friendly than she could really feel. One of them might one day become her daughter-in-law, and it would be pleasant if there had been only sweetness and understanding from the first, with none of the tart remarks and tactless reminiscences that she had suffered herself from both of her own mothers-in-law. She had tried to seem enough interested, but not too much. Too often—had she known—she praised to Tom the one before the last.

Prue—it surely was?—now leaned forward and in a low, confid-ing voice, admired the size of Kate's feet. 'And why do all of us young people have such enormous ones?' she lamented. 'I could never, never, wear shoes like those. Doesn't Lou despair, too?'

Louisa was more inclined to blame than to despair. 'They must have come from *somewhere*,' she had once said crossly, glaring at her feet in school walking-shoes, size seven. 'They must be somewhere in the family. Great feet like these don't come suddenly out of the blue. Unless you gave me the wrong kind of food when I was young.'

'Blue suits you so,' Prue now said.

'They condescend,' Kate thought. 'They behave like people who are trying hard not to be snobbish, and are led by that desire into an excess of insincerity. They are appalled for us that we are middle-aged.' She could remember trying to protect her own parents from the fact that their lives were virtually over.

She supposed blue did suit her, she agreed vaguely, to add something to the conversation; but talk about clothes bored her. It was like talk about sex. It had an enervating quality which had nothing to do with the subject itself.

'How is Lou?'

The girl had at last done with buttons and hemlines and whether she preferred chinchilla to mink.

'Very well,' said Kate. 'Home yesterday for the holidays.'

'You soon left her to her own devices. Good for you.'

'I had some important business.' Kate tried to keep frostiness out of her voice. She thought that the girl's efforts to be comradely were leading to awkwardness. Yes, Tom was well, too, she said in answer to the next question. 'Busy, though,' she added, anxious to spare, since Prue might have been wondering, these last few weeks, if the telephone would ever ring for her again. 'He's been helping Dermot to saw up great stacks of wood.' And also, she thought to herself, driving about the countryside until all hours with a lank-haired Spanish girl called Ignazia—as this poor young creature probably knew.

'Ignazia, what a frightening name,' she thought, turning to look out of her window, hoping for a pause, a rest. She had so often tried to imagine Tom's wedding and it had always been a local affair, the sort of wedding Lou would one day have, at the village church, but with the marquee in someone else's garden. As Prue had succeeded Susan, who succeeded Jane, Kate simply changed one sweet, pink, English face for another, and shifted the marquee into another garden. Now, all of a sudden, she was obliged to picture herself in Spain, with people crossing a great, cobbled square to the Cathedral. Tom would have changed his religion, if he still had one to change, and none of her friends would be there.

Perhaps Tom found these English girls insipid. 'Pink and white nullifidians'—wasn't that George Eliot's expression for them? she wondered. They were born to bloom under bridal veils, these girls—and all would, no doubt, in spite of Tom: and in no time at all, the bitter winds at point-to-points would break the veins on their cheeks, gardening would ruin their hands and the children's illnesses would line their foreheads. The size of their feet would be the least of their worries and it would seem long, long ago to them that they went to London to their secretarial colleges and wore those carefully chosen clothes and broke their hearts for love.

The train stopped at the station before Kate's and out poured the black business men on to the platform. They greeted one another briefly at the ticket-barrier and hurried up the slope towards the line of waiting cars, where their wives, who had rushed out in the middle of peeling potatoes or weeding rockeries, were waiting for them, with their thoughts all back at home where telephones might be ringing or children in mischief or things in saucepans boiling over the stove.

Was it what life should be? Kate wondered. It seemed so very little, although this girl sitting opposite her—she had forgotten her name again—was clearly desperate to achieve it, was now dabbing her face with powder as part of the campaign.

They came to the last familiar sequence of fields and copses. Such countless times Kate had looked out at them as the train slowed. The feeling that home was in the offing stirred her always, for she was not dulled by the habit of this journey as were those who came and went daily. Looking out, waiting, she checked the landmarks. The hedged lane ran under the bridge. Driving along it, the children had always shouted for her to sound the horn under the brick railway arch, loving to hear the echo, but that was years ago.

Kate knew the names of the houses now. Embowered in budding trees they lay on either side of the line among fields, houses where she had been to parties, those edge-of-the-country gatherings. The white house with green shutters had been her friend's, Dorothea's—no party place, that; but one where they had dined, together, the four of them, Dorothea bringing in the dishes herself, and, sometimes on Sunday evenings, supper on trays before the fire. The kitchen had been somewhere to drop into at any time when she needed an ear for anxieties about Tom or Louisa or for some improbable, absurd village story. And that was all in the past, too. Dorothea had died, and Kate saw now that she had relied on that friendship too much and was lost without it; she always averted her eyes from the house, shut up now and full of dust sheets, with the poor widower and his daughter both abroad.

Telling the fields over to herself, as if they were a charm, she had forgotten Prue. She knew who owned each of them, whose cows grazed in them, and which piece of land was next to be sold— regrettably—for building. The signal-box slid by and then the platform shelter threw its shadow into the carriages and the train stopped. More business men jumped out and hastened to the barrier, as if one moment would make all the difference.

'Good-bye, Mrs Heron,' Prue was saying. 'Do please give my love to Lou and everyone.'

'Yes, of course,' Kate murmured. 'Good-bye, my dear.' She would have added some message from herself, if she could have been sure enough who the girl was.

Beyond the barrier, Dermot was waiting.

.   .   .   .   .

'Ethel and her 'cello,' Dermot said, as they came out of the garage. 'I always thought it would make a nice title for a story.'

On this first sunny evening of the year, the house had all its windows thrown open, as if of itself, like a flower, it had responded to the sun. The sound of the 'cello—and of Louisa's effort to catch up with it on the piano—came clearly across the lawn. In the last bar, they were—by the skin of their teeth, Dermot said—united. The bow slurred across the strings, hanging on for Lou's last chord, seven notes down at once and three of them wrong ones. 'Oh, sorry. Damn,' she shouted and laughed and slammed down the piano lid.

'You see, I tied up the roses,' Dermot said.

The house was early Victorian and once had been a Vicarage. In the summer, white jasmine made the dark flint walls less gloomy. Kate, though, loved it as it was, at any time. The village lay in commuting country—an hour from London—and most of her friends lived in six-bedroomed villas, built twenty or thirty years ago in what she called Underwriters' Georgian. They had gardens full of flowering trees, bright gravel drives and tennis courts. The Old Vicarage had no flowering trees and hardly any flowers, but a shrubbery full of dark evergreens, plain lawns, a Wellingtonia, which was a landmark for miles, and a monkey-puzzle tree. Any plants that grew there had been put in years ago. The roses Dermot had tied up were plum-coloured and soft-petalled; though smelling sweet, they disintegrated at a touch and briars were growing from them. The moss-roses by the summer-house were turning into dog-roses.

Alan, Kate's first husband, had, though much disliking doing so, sometimes attempted a little pruning, but he had never been ruthless enough. Dermot cared only for chopping down trees or mowing the grass at a great pace or—at present—trying to grow mushrooms in an outhouse. This experiment, like others he had made, was going wrong in an undiagnosed way. Something should have happened by now, he told Kate, as he pushed the front door open for her, and then was irritated by her motherly smile. From the beginning she had treated the scheme as if it were child's play.

Louisa was crossing the hall.

'Oh, hello, Mummy,' she said, imitating a despised cousin. She

23

smiled and showed most of her teeth, looking bright and in-gratiating, cruelly Cynthia-like. 'Oh, hello, Daddy,' she said, turning the appalling smile on Dermot, who said, 'Out of my way, girl,' and went upstairs.

In the kitchen Mrs Meacock had pinned a folded napkin round her head as if she were a Stilton cheese and was singing as she popped a glacé cherry on top of each glassful of . . . whatever it was, Kate couldn't guess—one of the whips or mousses or soufflés she had learnt from the Americans she had last worked for and who had influenced her so much that it was rare for a dish of meat to go to the dining-room without its rings of tinned pineapple.

When she had finished with the cherries, instead of licking her fingers as she did when she was alone, she rinsed them under the tap and dried her hands carefully on the roller-towel. Little gusts of song were shaken from her.

'A lovely smell of mint,' said Kate, lifting the lid off the saucepan of potatoes.

'It makes all the difference in the world,' said Mrs Meacock. 'Although the O'Hogans preferred a dusting of carraway seeds. Not that they were very great potato eaters. And what was London like today?' she asked, as if she were enquiring after an invalid.

'Oh—the trees coming out, rather pretty, and warm. And did you have a good day? Did you get on with your book?'

It was not reading she was referring to, but compiling. Mrs Meacock was, like a bird building a nest, gathering material, sorting, putting together. Snippets from newspapers, quotations copied from library books, anecdotes from other people's anthologies filled a great many notebooks and cardboard boxes in her bedroom. 'Five Thousand and One Witty and Humorous Sayings,' as the book was to be called, was still a tangle of unrelated matter. On most afternoons she spent an hour unravelling it.

'I was going through some of the early ones,' she told Kate. 'It must have been twenty years ago I started collecting. When I first went into service with Mrs Lazenby. *He* used to write for *Punch*, I must have told you. Some of those early ones made me smile. I'd quite forgotten.'

So she had had a busy, happy afternoon, thought Kate. She seemed such a contented woman, dividing her enthusiasm between puddings and literary work.

Through the open window, she could hear Tom and Dermot talking on the path outside. 'I don't know how you stand it,' Dermot said. 'I should want to know who my master was.'

'He mustn't say such things,' Kate thought, glancing up quickly. Tom was muttering and scuffling the gravel, as he and his step-father went round the house.

Mrs Meacock gave the potatoes a prod and then began to strain them.

'I hope you found Mrs Heron Senior well,' she said through the steam. 'Not that I'd care twopence if she dropped down dead,' she thought.

.   .   .   .   .

Aunt Ethel descended the stairs wearing her beaded jersey and a touch of white talcum powder on her nose and cheekbones—a concession she made in the evenings. She had the ample, maternal, bosomy looks to be found in so many elderly spinsters. 'My children are scattered all over the world,' she sometimes told people, who did not always know that she referred to several hundred schoolgirls she had once taught.

Kate was coming out of the kitchen, so it was all right, Ethel thought, to make for the drawing-room, a place she avoided at this time of the evening if husband and wife were there alone together. Living in her niece's house involved her in all sorts of problems that no one else knew existed, and her habit of making herself scarce was noticed by no one but Dermot, who had been a parasite himself—and still was, some people thought. Ethel had a way of bending her head at closed doors, not listening, as she told herself, but ascertaining.

This evening, the drawing-room door was wide open. Within lay Tom upon the sofa. There was a glass of something on the table beside him and he was reading the back page of an evening paper. Louisa stood over the gramophone with a record in her hand and Ethel was sorry to see this. It would be jazz, she thought. All popular tunes she called jazz. The moment the noise began, brother and sister, silent hitherto, would start a conversation. When this happened, she clapped her hands over her ears in what she hoped was a mock protest. If she had not been living under their mother's roof, she would have been more pointed.

Tom, seeing her, half-heartedly swung his legs off the sofa and dropped his newspaper, and Ethel put up her hand and shook her head as if to stop him disturbing himself more—which he really had no intention of doing, as she knew.

'Do you hate this row?' Lou shouted.

'I'll bet it's not half as jolly as the tunes she had when she was young,' Tom said, lifting the newspaper as a screen and knowing only his sister could hear him. 'Trot here, trot there,' he began to warble against the sound of the record. 'That's my favourite. *Véronique*, isn't it? Very catchy.'

'I really neither hate nor like it,' Ethel told Lou. 'It just doesn't seem nearly as jolly as the tunes we had when I was a girl.'

'Mother says we have all the same tunes, but not played so well,' Lou said.

'The singers seem less successful in love than they used to be. So full of self-pity. Faint heart never won fair lady.'

'Don't you think it would be a good idea, Tom,' said Dermot, coming in with some ice in a bowl, 'if you bestirred yourself and saw that Ethel was comfy?'

'Here,' said Tom quickly, entangling himself in newspaper. 'Come and be comfy here, Auntie, on the sofa.'

'Now don't put yourself out, dear boy. That was naughty of you, Dermot. There are all these other chairs in the room.'

'I was brought up to stand when ladies came in,' Dermot said, using unconsciously an old-fashioned Irish voice.

Lou flushed and said, 'And so was Tom. He only forgot.'

'And you will pardon my chivvying you, Tom. I should like some lemon for Mum's drink. Did your horse win?'

'I didn't *have* a horse.'

'Are you sure you don't mind this row?' Lou shouted at her aunt. 'Mum, do you mind this row?' she repeated, as Kate came in.

'Perhaps a little quieter . . .'

'Tom's fetching some lemon,' Dermot said.

'Perhaps when this one comes to the end, Lou, that *could* be the end.'

'You don't really like it, do you?'

'Not if you don't want me to. I just marvel at the tune's having lasted all these years.'

'Imperishable stuff,' said Dermot.

She looked at him quickly, wondering if he were teasing her, as the children did. She had always to pause before she could remember what the world was like when he was young. In age, he was almost as near to Tom as he was to her: in outlook, much nearer. There were three distinct generations in the house—her Aunt Ethel's, then her own, and her children's. Between hers and Tom's and Lou's, on the mezzanine floor as it were, was Dermot's.

Tom had come back with the lemon and he decorated her drink and handed it to her.

Aunt Ethel began to make protestations to Dermot: first, that she would have nothing to drink; then came a long story about how she had had some sherry a fortnight ago and had felt muzzy afterwards; of course, if she *were* to have anything, it must not be spirits, for she did not think—speaking only for herself—that spirits did any good to the liver. At last, she hit on the one thing Dermot could not find. Tom, looking martyred, went to search for Dubonnet. 'Campari,' Dermot suggested, when no Dubonnet could be found. 'This you'll enjoy, I know.' He could not endure to wait any longer for his own drink.

'Then truly only the tiniest drop. And now I must remember not to have my tot at bedtime. No, that's far too much, you know. I shall be tipsy.'

'Try hard,' said Dermot. 'Anything, Lou?'

'I don't drink.'

'It's rather bitter, isn't it?' asked Ethel, pressing her lips together and shuddering.

Dermot had scarcely poured his own drink when he was back among the bottles to refill his glass. Kate watched Tom moving over to the table to join him. 'Your new husband is a bad example to us young lads,' he had once told her. His joke, like so many others that he made, induced shame and anxiety. Prepared at first to feel like Hamlet's mother, ready for bitter jealousies and resentments, she was bewildered to find the reverse of those things, an extraordinary and unlooked-for affection and admiration of Hamlet for Claudius—allies at race-meetings, leaning over bars, laughing at their betters, as they called it, they seemed, but for the worship on one side, much the same age. Alan, who had never been to a race-meeting in his life and drank in dining-rooms or hardly at all, would have worried, and Kate, for all her explaining to herself that Tom was twenty-two now, worried too.

'Ah, you old duffer,' Ethel shouted as her dog came skidding across the polished floor towards her.

'What's he been rolling in *now*?' Tom asked, bunching his handkerchief up before his nose.

'Punch! What a nasty smell,' Ethel said fondly and patted her lap. Up lumbered the aged spaniel to have the dead leaves collected from his coat.

'The Castle's come back,' Lou said. She had taken up Alan's old telescope which was kept by the south window for looking at the view. As she tried to focus it, the wavering blur of green and blue suddenly sharpened and she could see the Thames Valley lying below, with wooded hillsides and orchards, roof-tops, in the distance the gas-holder at Staines, the grand-stand at Ascot and, with the setting sun striking the tops of towers and ramparts, the Castle itself, set high against the horizon.

'Come and see, Aunt Ethel. It's the first time this year that it's come out of the mist.'

'I can see it with my naked eyes,' Tom said, glancing briefly. Royalty, and where they lived, bored him.

'But not the windows and the flag.'

Aunt Ethel put Punch down and took her stand behind the telescope.

'The View,' Kate said, smiling at Dermot.

Evening after evening, year after year, the family was drawn to it, visitors were always required to look and admire and have the landmarks pointed out to them—the War Memorial at Runnymede, the Hog's Back near Guildford. Alan had been rather pompous about it—'our view', sometimes 'my view'. When they were young, he had lifted the children on to the window-sill and held the telescope steady for them, focusing it patiently, Lou excitedly exclaiming at what she saw; first, perhaps, a branch of lilac, and a bird very large in the foreground, and then—she would sigh with enchantment—the grey or white or golden castle where the Princesses lived. 'Yes, I can see all right,' Tom would say, looking briefly at a vista; whether blurred or otherwise, he was bored with it. They were a different family then and Dermot not a part of it.

Now Dermot smiled back at Kate. The view had become a joke to him even before he was married to her, when he had been a guest in this room. And he had laughed at many another solemn ritual, broken through imprisoning habits, not questioning who had begun them, or how they had gained their hold, and he had earned Tom's gratitude and been resented by Lou, who was not quite ready to be set free.

At this time of evening, Kate felt that he was restless. He had had too many years of pubs and clubs and pleasing himself. Not to be free to walk out of the house when he wanted to must seem a monstrous tyranny. She, herself, sometimes in the course of this second marriage, found it a tyranny, too; found other people's presence irksome.

'The cherry orchards are coming into blossom,' Lou announced, having taken her turn again with the telescope.

'After supper, shall we go for a drive?' Kate asked Dermot. Sooner or later, she had to be alone with him and talk about his mother. It would be worse if he thought she had put this off or been reluctant.

'We could go over to The George and Dragon,' he said, looking much brighter.

Though he was always kind and thoughtful to Aunt Ethel, Kate knew that some of the evenings in her company, the hour or two after supper, drove him to the edge of frenzy.

She guessed that he must have heard the kitchen door opening as well as she had. Pretending that he had no idea that supper was imminent he poured out a drink for himself.

'Right you are, then,' said Mrs Meacock, popping her head round the door. This meant that the cutlets and the stuffed tomatoes that the American family had liked so much, were ready.

.   .   .   .   .

As soon as she was alone with Dermot after dinner, Kate realised how cleverly she must put her sentences together; tactful phrases must seem careless, but the carelessness must not verge on indifference or she would be accused of condescending. This had happened soon after their marriage, when one of Dermot's many precarious and temporary jobs had come to a sudden end. Less skilled than she now was, she had hoped to save his pride by making little of the matter. 'So it's of no importance whether I work or not?' he had asked her. 'Perhaps you were thinking all along that so little money was not worth bothering about.' She knew that the argument might just as well have gone the other way; that, no matter what she said, her words would be like sparks in a dry thicket.

She was glad that it was dark as they drove riverwards to The George and Dragon. She had only her voice to manage, lightly (she hoped) describing the day's happenings. Dermot, edgily, was waiting. He was beginning to wonder if she would ever speak and was searching for some question to ask her. No doubt words would be said which he would much rather not have to listen to;

30

but the sooner they were out, the sooner he could begin to recover from them. Between the two of them the tension gathered, and Kate found herself counting, as if she were dropping in a parachute.

'What did you have for lunch?' Dermot asked at last.

'Fricassee of chicken.'

'Nice?'

'Very.'

He changed gear and began to whistle softly. 'Good,' he said presently. 'How are things at Harrods?'

'Simply splendid. In fact, we talked about shops a great deal—your mother says Lord Auden's going to have one now—Victorian junk. Edwina is quite excited.'

'Is she going to serve in it? I can see the two of them being gracious and gay and giving the wrong change. I wonder what my father would have said.'

'She had it in mind for you to do those things. I doubt if she will broach the matter again, but if she does I hope you will keep a straight face.'

'Did *you*?'

'Yes.'

She was quiet and wary and afraid of disturbing his anger.

'How dare they discuss me when I'm not there,' he thought. Kate was as much to blame as his mother in his mind. He might have been a child. Their ridiculous schemes humiliated him so much that every word in which they spoke of them left its scar. He could not risk more, fearing to hear something too monstrous, something from which his resilient self-respect would never recover, which would separate him from Kate, whom he so deeply loved.

His love for her was his chief pride. Throughout his life, dissolving affections, the most fleeting sensations of tenderness, had left him immune. His heart had been even more resilient than his self-respect. From broken affairs he rapidly recovered without convalescence. They left no blank and sometimes he was sorry that they did not, thinking himself deprived of what other people had and seemed to value, though it caused them grief, and anxiety. Until he met Kate and began rather gradually and unsuspectingly to love her, he had never known anxiety. Now he was afraid of happenings from which he would not recover.

'I could do with a drink,' he said crossly.

'Well, we are nearly there.'

He heard Kate's sigh. Hastily, before he pulled the blind down for ever over Lord Auden's shop-window, he said: 'Poor mother, she has always been hare-brained.'

'So amusing, though,' Kate replied.

She was always conscious of a change in Dermot's manner when he stepped across the threshold of a public house. 'Seize hope, all ye who enter here,' might have been written above the porch, and he could hardly wait to open the door and urge her forwards into the hubbub.

Across the room, where horse-brasses and copper skillets framed the fireplace, Kate was sorry to see four of her acquaintances—middle-aged couples who had been in the background of her life with Alan. They had met at other people's parties or on the London train; one pair had sometimes played golf with Alan; both had sent wreaths when he died. After the letters of sympathy and the flowers, Kate heard nothing from them.

Dermot, however, had, it now appeared, met one of the husbands—Harry. They had a special Sunday lunch-time place which had exactly the right kind of beer for that time of the morning of that day of the week. From these jaunts Dermot—Tom often accompanying him—would return late, upsetting Mrs Meacock. Harry's wife was none too pleased, either, it seemed, for with what she obviously thought was delicate raillery and everyone else took for justifiable though embarrassing irritation, she began, as soon as she saw Dermot, to accuse him of keeping her husband from his luncheon. There was a long plaint about roast beef dried up and Yorkshire puddings fallen flat and of afternoons through which Harry dozed and snored, covered in newspaper. Wasn't it too bad, she asked Kate, who smiled, but would not offer Mrs Meacock and many an overdone sirloin in exchange. Harry looked shamed and everyone else looked bored, but it was difficult—so settled to her denunciations his wife was—to make any change in the conversation.

Not actually listening to Mrs Harry—Myra was her name, she remembered—Kate tried to seem as if she were, and then found herself looking too fixedly at the woman's face. Under this concentrated gaze, Myra faltered, lost the thread of what she was saying and, taking a mirror from her handbag, glanced at it anxiously.

The others had moved a little away and were arguing about politics. Dermot's voice had its Abbey Theatre intonation—a sign of crisis, Kate knew; either in love or dissension.

All the exasperation he had felt—with his mother, Lord Auden, himself, the mushrooms that would not grow—he now decided had come from none of those sources, but from the government's inability to put an end to a strike of fish-porters.

'I know nothing about politics,' he kept saying, 'but I know *this* much.' What was the government to do, Harry wondered. Bring in the troops?

'Take a strong line,' said Dermot, finishing off his glass of whisky. He had the utmost confidence in his view of the matter, of the wrongness of all the Nonconformist porters who were preventing decent Roman Catholics from having their fish on Fridays. Religious feeling came in with the Irish accent, was put on quickly like a false moustache.

Kate, listening, would rather they had all gone on talking about Yorkshire puddings. Dermot, who had had too much gin before dinner and too much whisky since, was becoming muddled. There occurred a dangerous moment when, like a bull barbed and defeated and with escape cut off, he was confronted by his own earlier remarks, quoted by Harry to vanquish him. His fine denunciation had gone on some way since then and somehow altered its course; and Harry's quotations muddled him and made him suspicious, seeming to be the reverse of what he was now trying to prove. Worse than having destroyed his case was the realisation that he had brought himself and his opponents (too late now for them to draw back as, for Kate's sake, they wished to do) to the position where he was most vulnerable. He wondered how he could have been so foolish as to begin an argument which had the possibility of taking such a turn. From the subject of strikes—'crippling the country,' he said, 'strangling economy and holding a gun to our heads'—it was a short step to denouncing those who did not want to work, and there they were, all miserably embarrassed, at Dermot Heron, who threw up every job after a week or two and lately had not even tried to start one.

Kate knew the silence was coming and, when it did, the awkwardness of it froze her heart. Dermot broke it, saying that they all talked too much, though he more than any, he admitted. He thought that he saw Harry smile at Myra and guessed that the smile had been returned and understood. Turning, half against his will, to make sure, he was checked by the sight of Kate, who was gazing at a row of bottles behind the bar, pretending to have heard nothing.

'Nothing happened,' she was thinking. 'Nothing was said. But one day, in this or other country, it *will* be said.' It was a great relief to be spared it for the present. She felt drained of strength and patience and was suffering the boredom for which she would later be blamed.

On the way home they quarrelled—or, rather, she listened to Dermot quarrelling with an imaginary Kate, who supplied him with imaginary retorts, against which he was able to build up his indignation. Then, when they were nearly home, he began to punish himself, and Kate realised that the more he basked in blame, the more it would turn out to be all hers; her friends, for close friends of hers they would become, would seem to have lined up to aggravate him, and her silence would be held to account for his lack of it.

'And who for God's sake does Harry think he is?' Dermot asked. 'Trundling back and forth to London day after day. And

34

poor little Myra, with her pinched-up face and that frightened laugh—unhappy creature, scared of the dull oaf. She has worn herself out with her own nagging. They are all the most contemptible bunch of middle-aged, middle-class commuting jackasses.'

My friends, thought Kate. And Alan's.

'I know they're your friends,' he said, 'and I take off my hat to you for enduring them all these years, but *I* can't endure them, I'm afraid.'

'You couldn't know that they would be in the pub,' Kate said, with deceptive gentleness.

In the old days, Alan, when he had trundled back from London, had been tired. After dinner he played Beethoven quartets on the gramophone, and dozed. Some evenings, Kate, having written her letters to the children at school, became restless. Nowadays, there was no chance of being restless, just as there were no more Beethoven quartets. Only Tom and Louise played the gramophone. No one had touched Alan's records since he died. Dermot, picking his way round Kate's remark, suspecting some criticism of himself, said: 'I thought it was you who suggested coming out. If you didn't want to go to The George and Dragon, I wish that you had said so. I thought you looked so bored the last time we went to The Spread Eagle, and you say it's too stuffy at The Bird In Hand. I think it's you who is being difficult, you know. Darling Kate,' he added.

'One place is much the same as another, I dare say,' she said, soothingly, as if he were a fretful child. 'And I said before, you couldn't know that Harry would be there.'

'I would rather you stabbed me in the back than condescended to me.'

'I'm not given to stabbing people in the back.'

'No, you are different from your friends.'

She could not keep up with him. He swung from one subject to another, like a monkey in a tree, so she leant back and shut her eyes and let him go through his antics on his own.

He was like this when she first came to know him, she reminded herself, and when she married him she was too old to believe in schemes for changing him or bending him to a more amenable pattern. That people can change—sometimes even violently—she had realised, but if Dermot ever did so he would become a different person, and she could not imagine him different. She had married him as he was and would do so again now, she knew, and at any time in the future.

'I'm sorry if I ruined your evening,' he said, shaving past Tom's car as he drove into the garage. 'I won't talk so much in future.' Once he could get over the wretched, uncomfortable present, he was sure of managing the future very well indeed.

Everyone was in bed. Aunt Ethel had done her usual tidying up, had emptied the ash-trays and put away bottles, taken *The Times* from a waste-paper basket and gone upstairs to read it. 'I never touch it until everyone else has finished with it,' she often explained.

From Tom's room came the sound of dance music on his wireless. 'They *are* the same tunes as we had when I was young,' Kate said. Seeing the light shining under Louisa's door, she tapped gently and went in.

Lou was sitting up in bed, writing, with her hand curved protectingly round the page. She looked up at Kate expectantly, waiting—probably—for her to go away again. In the striped pyjamas she insisted on wearing and with her hair brushed down straight to her shoulders, she looked like a little girl, no more than twelve years old.

'It's so lovely to have you home,' Kate said.

'Lovely to *be* here,' Lou replied, 'and have a comfortable bed again.' Yet, already, the privacy was palling. She missed the dormitory chatter—the secrets, the conspiracy—and the company of those who laid no burdens on her if she loved them, to whom she could give her affection as she chose and withdraw it again when she pleased. She hated school, she thought, but missed it when she was at home.

Her bedroom was untidy. Still waiting to be put away were heaps of books and clothes. Her father's photograph—the only one on show in the house—aloofly surveyed the confusion.

'You will get it all straight tomorrow, won't you?' Kate said, bending to kiss her.

The hand spread over the page, the girl's wide gaze held her off and Kate felt rebuffed, as if she were thought untrustworthy.

Lou smelt of toothpaste and her hair was cool and silky against Kate's cheek.

'Don't leave your light on too long.' Kate was always, like most mothers, wasting words and knowing she wasted them.

'It can't be anything but painful, having daughters,' she thought, closing the door. 'Wanting so much for them, and dreading so much, yet unable to ensure or prevent a thing. One is quite useless.'

.   .   .   .

Aunt Ethel's room had once been a nursery and the windows were still barred. Before one of these she now stood in the moonlight, doing her breathing exercises. Her stout figure in mannish pyjamas looked like a Teddy bear's, her feet were planted widely apart and her arms rose and fell stiffly. Then she drew the curtains across and switched on the light. The room did not spring to life at once. So dense with furniture was it, so littered with possessions, that the light seemed to pick out one piece after another. It was as if an oil lamp were gaining strength, striking the gilt harp first, then the cheval looking-glass, until at last everything—the ivory-handled button-hook, unused for fifty years, the pin-cushion, the ring stand, dumb-bells, rowing machine, each photograph—stood clear.

Every evening Ethel struggled upstairs with her 'cello and the music-stand, for it was a part of the parasite's code not to litter up other people's houses with one's things. 'I never leave anything lying about,' she would tell visitors. 'Kate's very good and I wouldn't take advantage of her for the world.'

Before she got into bed, she swallowed some pills containing desiccated liver and garlic and then she began to beat some

37

petroleum jelly into her weathered cheeks. God helps those who help themselves, was her belief. In any pause during the day, when other people might have lit a cigarette, she could be seen with a glass of water in one hand and half a dozen pills in the other, her eyes glazed and staring as she swallowed. 'It must cost a fortune,' Dermot would say. 'Though I must say it seems to be worth it. Anyone might take you for my daughter.'

To this there would be some tart reply, but she would keep his remark in mind for later and bring it out in the solitude of her bedroom and enjoy it privately, like a biscuit saved from tea.

.   .   .   .   .

Dermot was staring at his face in the looking-glass as Kate came into the bedroom.

'Shall I grow a moustache?' he asked—to imply that this was all he had been considering.

Some tablets were fizzing in a glass of water on the dressing-table. He watched them dissolve, then swallowed them.

His drinking evenings had the same pattern always, as she knew. Caution, exhilaration, aggressiveness were followed by the diminuendo of face-saving, self-reproach, reproach, attempts at recovery, back to caution again.

She began to undress. She was tired and luncheon with Edwina seemed a week ago. When she was depressed, she could not help reflecting on the hazards of having married a husband so much younger than herself. Her fear that he should ever regret doing so shadowed her self-confidence. For a while, she had even been tempted to try to appear much younger than she was, but early recognised this for the trap it must always be. Now Dermot, for his part, seemed to be doing his best to catch up with her; his handsome features had become less defined and his thick, wavy hair had begun to recede. This had caused his mother, on her last visit, great distress, and she had come as near as she dared—and was a woman who dared a great deal—to suggesting that Kate was to blame for the onset of baldness, as she was for a missing button on his coat sleeve. 'He was so fussy about his clothes,' she said.

Standing in the middle of the bedroom in socks and crumpled shirt, drinking his fizzy drink, he must be, Kate thought, the opposite of the picture in his mother's imagination.

'I wish Edwina could see you now,' she told him.

'I suppose I take after my father,' Dermot said, swallowing the last of his drink, looking preoccupied, because full of wind. 'He had his shoe-laces ironed and his pocket-linings taken out and laundered every week. That's better. I feel better now. Excuse me. In fact, Father was nothing *but* clothes; the suits were more him than he was himself. When I opened his wardrobe after he died, I thought, "There's poor old Patrick after all, so what's the fuss been all about?" I couldn't think why my mother was so put out. She had married a very fine morning-suit and there it still was in a moth-proof bag. Now, you, on the contrary,' he said, throwing his socks across the room, 'look at this moment as if you had never worn a stitch in all your life, never covered yourself up from the weather; brown all the year round and smelling of fresh air.'

Will-power and his pride with, perhaps, the help of the fizzy drink, on whose magic he so touchingly depended, had repaired his disorder. He could have walked along a chalked line or recited Gray's 'Elegy' by heart. Only the indiscretion in the pub remained to rankle. He would make love to her and fall asleep in her arms and then wake in the night to remember his disgrace and make once more his vows about drinking. In the middle of the night, the vows were easily and often made.

'What is more,' he said, 'you look as if you have been polished. Once upon a time, I had a rich acquaintance who had a bronze statue in his hall—a naiad or however you pronounce it, with lovely buttocks like yours, *clenched* like that.' He shook his fist at her. 'One day, when I was passing by, I suddenly couldn't resist them. I fought my way through the potted palms and began to stroke her behind, this naiad's. Luckily, it was Derby Day.'

'Why luckily?'

'Well, all the time and unbeknown to me the butler was watching. When I turned round, he was standing there, looking scared, trying to put the unperturbed expression back on his face. I might have been at a loss for words at any other time, but not then. "Never Say Die is what you want for the big race," I said, as quick as a flash, and "Thank you, sir," said he.'

'And did it win?' asked Kate, putting her arms fast round him as he got into bed.

'It romped all the way home like a child off to a party.'

He ran his knuckles down her spine. 'You taste of rain,' he said, kissing her. 'People say I married her for her money,' he thought contentedly, and for the moment was full of the self-respect that loving her had given him.

[2]

AUNT ETHEL came into her own at breakfast-time for, since her second marriage, as part of the general demoralisation (Ethel thought), Kate had taken to having hers in bed. Dermot always wandered about the room while she did so, still wearing his pyjamas, reading sheets of the newspaper which were spread in disorder over the eiderdown and going over to Kate's tray from time to time to butter a slice of toast for himself. For some reason he liked to tell people that he did not have breakfast. This morning, he felt wonderfully healthy again, and full of energy. He had been a little queasy when he awoke, but toast and honey soon put him right.

Ethel ate honey, too. 'The Ancient Greeks trained on it for the Olympic Games,' she told Tom, who had been told before. He and Lou sat on either side of her and this allowed her a motherly attitude towards them, which she could not have assumed at any other time of the day.

Tom was reading the back page of a newspaper and Lou leant across the table to peer at the headlines on the front.

'What a horrible world,' she said. 'It's like the Middle Ages, all dark and smelling of blood. I wonder if I shall be lucky enough to see thirty.'

'Nonsense, child,' said Ethel, 'it's an age of illimitable scope and possibility. Even in my lifetime, people may go to the moon.'

'I am frightened enough already, without bringing the moon into it. It's no wonder that young men like Tom care only for today and become juvenile delinquents and drug themselves with trivial things, such as horse-racing.'

Tom raised his eyes from the day's runners and looked suspiciously at his sister.

'What you need, Louisa,' Ethel said, 'is a course of Vitamin B. You sound rather sorry for yourself. I expect you've been working too hard.'

'Better have some honey,' Tom said. 'I suppose I must go to work. He swears more about my being a couple of minutes late than he would if all the rest came in at ten o'clock. You'd think it would be the other way round—I being his grandson. "What about blood being thicker than water?" I feel like saying. "Poor Father," I think all day long. Fancy having him about the place all the time he was young. No wonder he wouldn't go into the business when he grew up.'

'You're lucky to have it there to step into,' Ethel said. 'And your grandfather is strict with you, because he wants to leave it in good hands.'

'I hate self-made men. They think everyone else should slave as they have done. "You missed the lot," I'll say to him one day. "Grubbing about like that from morning to night, you never lived. What have you got?" I'll say—"a great stack of money, a knighthood, the respect of your competitors, and that's about the lot. Not a moment's fun have you had. No one's ever been really pleased to see you and no one will give a damn when you die." '

'I can hear you saying it,' said Lou.

'If you feel like that, you were wrong to take the job,' Ethel said.

'Tell me, what else could I do? I haven't Father's brains or his patience. I've a good mind to pack it in, though. Yes, I've a good mind to tell him so. I might go into the wine trade. Ignazia knows some importers. Sherry and so on. My God, how I loathe sherry.' He glanced again at the newspaper, scribbled something in his diary and got up. 'Could you press my trousers, Lou? I left them on the end of the bed. There's a kind sister.'

'It's strange,' Lou said slowly, when he had gone. 'Blood isn't really thicker than water. Don't you think Tom is much more like Dermot than our own father? All that about what he's going to tell people and never doing it. Going into the wine trade, indeed. That's Dermot all over.'

Ethel felt awkward at Lou's discernment.

'Perhaps we ought not to discuss people behind their backs,' she suggested.

'We can't very well discuss them in front of them,' said Lou.

'Tom seems discontented in his job. I had never imagined him cut out for that sort of thing. When he was a little boy, I sometimes thought he would be a great conductor. He was always beating time to music. At the kindergarten, he played the cymbals in their little percussion band and I used to watch him at the end-of-term concerts and think how much more idea of it he had than the other children. After all, there is music in the family. Your Uncle Jack played the fiddle.'

'And you with your 'cello,' Lou said kindly.

'Ah well, I've no illusions that that gives pleasure to anyone but me. All the same . . .'

'What did you imagine me becoming?' 'A mother, I expect,' Lou thought.

'As a matter of fact, I used to listen to you questioning people about things . . . always so alert . . . you wouldn't be fobbed off or coaxed away from a subject. "With that sort of mind she could go anywhere," I thought. "Perhaps be England's first woman judge. How splendid that would be," I used to think. I could see you as plainly as this pot of honey, togged up in your robes and wearing a wig and going at the head of a procession to open the Assizes. Just like a picture.'

'How disappointingly we grew up,' Lou said, with a false sigh.

.   .   .   .   .

Kate leant back against the pillows reading her letters and yawning. She had wakened before daybreak and lain worrying about Dermot and the children's future. She had told herself that as soon as morning came the troubles would appear surmountable, but this did not stop her from continuing to fret, even about quite trivial things. In the darkness she heard the first note from a bird, far away by the river, and then the chorus gathered, growing in volume it filled the Thames Valley, was handed on from branch to branch, up the wooded hillsides, till all the birds in the world seemed to be in a frenzy, the birds in the churchyard and in all the cottage gardens and in the trees above Kate's bedroom window.

It is a callous hour. She remembered waking to it on the morning after Alan had died, becoming coldly conscious that she must begin her first day without him, and feeling sorry that she had slept at all, that someone from kindness had given her a draught—for the grief came fresh, nourished while she had slept, and the shock was to be suffered again. As indifferent to the silent house, the colourless sky, the chorusing of the birds had been—some too close, under the eaves, making what had seemed to her strident and spiteful noises. Then there had been, as there were this morning, those banal exchanges from tree to tree, mockings and bickerings and sudden solo trillings. When she was a child, allowed to sleep out-of-doors for a treat, she had sometimes wakened and thought that early-morning clamour the most enchanting sound in the world.

Now, at least it meant that the night was over. As the room grew lighter, she became more hopeful, and by the time she heard Mrs Meacock going downstairs her anxieties were beginning to seem trivial, the future was smoothed out. Tom might at last settle down to work and stop gambling and Dermot, if he could not go as far as to set a good example, might give up setting a bad one. Ignazia could at any time be recalled to Spain by an ailing parent; Lou would, without too much disturbance to herself, grow out of her religious phase. Kate's optimism now soared higher (she heard Aunt Ethel's bedroom door open) to the expectation of miracles—such as Dermot's finding the outhouse carpeted with mushrooms and Ethel marrying the Vicar and removing herself to the Vicarage.

Ethel had crossed the landing and tapped on Tom's door, for he must not be late for Sir Alfred. A smell of bacon frying came upstairs and Ethel's dog began to bark at the postman. Last of all in

44

the house to stir, Dermot had groaned and flung an arm across her pillow. Greeting the day with his usual brave resolve about temperance, he had struggled out of bed to make another fizzy drink.

Mrs Meacock had brought in the breakfast tray and the letters. There was one for Kate from Araminta, daughter of her friend Dorothea, who had died. That Tom and Araminta should one day marry had been their mothers' daydream, and still was Kate's.

'She is coming back from France,' she told Dermot, handing him the letter. 'She is opening up the house again ready for when Charles comes from Bahrain.'

'I suppose you are already sending Ignazia off with a flea in her ear,' he said. He was a long time reading the letter, frowning over a phrase or two the girl had written in French. 'I'm afraid I can only read simple things like "Arc de Triomphe",' he told Kate.

This was probably near the truth, she reflected. She was still often surprised by what Dermot did not know and it was a puzzle to her that he could have spent so many years at school and have so little to show for them. His handwriting was childish, his spelling eccentric, and when he played darts he could seldom subtract his score. All of his modest efforts to make money ended in confusions of figures from which he could only extricate the fact that he had less than he had when he started. The mushroom-growing would be the same, in spite of all the people he had heard about who had made so much money from similar schemes.

'Before Araminta comes, we might have a little holiday,' Kate said.

This sense of pleasurable anticipation would not have seemed possible to her an hour or so earlier that morning. 'It could be our honeymoon. We've never really had one.' Three days of love-making and drinking while the rain poured down the windows of their hotel in Cornwall she did not count.

'I thought we had a very nice honeymoon,' Dermot said. 'Are you going to eat that piece of toast? You're sure, now?' He was as anxiously insistent as if he were talking to a child. 'From ancient

45

times, the energy-giving properties of honey have been well known to man,' he said in Ethel's voice.

'It is good of you to put up with her,' Kate said, not for the first time.

'I don't put up with her, I like her.'

'She has nowhere else to go that wouldn't be intolerably dreary. And she was good to me when Alan died. I couldn't have said to her, "You've kept me company and filled the gap, but now that I've fallen in love, I want the house to myself again".'

'No, I can't hear you saying that,' said Dermot. With the faint stir of unease with which he saw anyone set off to work, he watched Tom going towards the garage.

'Is that Tom?' Kate asked, as she heard the doors grating on the gravel as they were pulled open. She glanced at the bedside clock and sighed.

'He's in plenty of time,' Dermot said.

'Only if he drives too fast.'

'What's five minutes, for heaven's sake? Surely the man doesn't build up a great crisis for that?'

'Tom's rebellious enough as it is, Dermot. Don't encourage him.'

'Good Lord, I don't encourage him.' Dermot turned away from the window and looked at her in surprise.

. . . . .

From her bedroom window, Ethel saw Dermot come out on to the gravel path and stand there hesitantly for a moment or two. The old gardener who came once a week was already at work in the vegetable plot beyond the currant bushes. Moving about among the plumy kale, he was dun-coloured, looked as friable as dry earth.

Dermot's manner, Ethel thought, was unlike that of the master of the house stepping outside to have a look at the garden after breakfast. He did not glance up at the sky or sniff the air or move forward to straighten the bent stake in the weedy border. He just stood there, looking idle and irresolute, as a guest might.

46

It was possible, Ethel decided, stepping back into the room and beginning to make her bed, that at this time of day, when their neighbours' cars were going by like shoals of fish, Dermot might feel conscious of not hurrying off to work himself. His usual discouraged look into the mushroom shed could hardly be called that.

Ethel's lips moved busily while she smoothed the sheets, and made what she called hospital corners. 'I will say that for myself,' she was thinking. 'I do know how to make a bed properly.'

When she peeped out of the window again, Dermot was still standing there, but, as if he became conscious of her looking down on him, he suddenly braced himself and walked away—towards the outhouses, she observed.

'I give this marriage five years at most,' she had written to her friend, Gertrude. 'Without being too brutal, one must admit that she has bought him for herself with the money Alan left her, and one day he, Dermot, will begin to find that being her property is irksome. Then, when the physical side grows less important, she may think she hasn't got her money's worth.'

When they met, Ethel and Gertrude often had straightforward talks about the 'physical side'. Neither had had any experience of it, but they had read a great deal about the matter—even manuals on the technique of sex, as they called it. Lacking photographs, these books were sometimes puzzling, and Ethel was inclined to imagine Dermot and her niece engaged in the most complicated acrobatics. None the less, unlimited though the variety of its expressions might be, sex was something which must—and Gertrude agreed—wear itself out. Of its very nature, they contended.

It seemed—and before Ethel expected—to have worn itself out already, or had worn Kate out first. Everything was too much for her, whether getting up for breakfast or seeing that Tom behaved himself. Dermot, for his part, was a minute or two earlier at the drinks tray every evening. Ethel sometimes found it difficult not to

47

look at her watch. She would not have accepted a drink herself before a quarter past seven, she said.

One of Ethel's greatest pleasures was letter-writing, and she looked forward to composing, later in the day, a long analysis of her niece's marriage to send to Gertrude. It would be as minutely observed as if she were Richard Jefferies describing a hedgerow. She would compare the second marriage with the first and give two contrasting pictures—the evening with Alan, listening to chamber music; the evenings now, tearing off to public houses or else going too early to bed.

'Not that I don't love Dermot very much,' she thought, and her lips moved and she shook her head. She went to the wash-basin and drank some water and swallowed two liver extract pills. 'I always have a good colour,' she thought and leaned close to the mirror to look at the confusions of broken veins on her cheeks.

    .   .   .   .   .

Louisa's bedroom was as cluttered as Ethel's, not with an accumulation of objects loved or necessary, but with things she had eagerly collected not very long ago and would soon discard. At school, she was making her mark as an eccentric, and the properties of her eccentricity were displayed about the room amidst the disorders of unpacking. A curled-up school photograph hung on one drawing-pin from a beam. 'All those busty girls,' Tom had said.

'What on earth do you want that pith helmet for, and that disgusting old ear-trumpet?' Kate had asked her.

'I should feel pretty silly without them,' Lou replied.

Her mother had also protested about the stolen notices, all forbidding something—trespassing, the sale of alcohol to persons under the age of eighteen, the passing of betting-slips.

'Well, I've got them now,' Lou said. 'I should look a proper fool trying to smuggle them back where they came from.'

'Yes, but do get rid of them. It looks so bad.'

'Mother, you don't understand the trouble I took getting them and all the risks I ran. "Penalty Five Pounds" I've promised to

Caroline Barlow anyway. I'll just keep the rest till I get tired of them. You know how soon I tire of things. And Dermot's just promised me a very special one from a gents' lavatory.'

'If you keep them you keep them against my wishes,' Kate said, now more aggravated by Dermot than Lou.

'Oh, *thank you*, Mother,' said Lou.

'Her moral attitude seems slightly hay-wire,' she had written about Kate in her diary that night. At school—though Lou disagreed with nearly everything they said—the mistresses seemed more consistent, as Alan, her father, had always been consistent.

At this age, Louisa found exasperating and rather humiliating the halting concessions which were made to her grown-upness and also the privileges half-given and then snatched back because of her adolescence. She would rather not have a glass of sherry at all, than have it offered suddenly one evening, as if a date on the calendar had been reached, when her constitution was judged able to withstand the shock of sudden alcohol. 'I don't drink,' she said then, and she had said so ever since, hoping to punish them with her abstemiousness. Who decided on those dates, she wondered, and made the rules for growing up? Dermot could bet on horses and talk about them constantly, but when Tom, ten years or so his junior, did so, his mother frowned and looked perturbed.

Just lately, Lou had decided that there must also be stages in Kate's own life, for until recently it had not been right, or had appeared not to be right, for her to do a great many things that she did now—playing darts in the village pub, going to race-meetings, having breakfast in bed, kissing her husband in public.

Though she treated Lou as a child about going to bed—not actually telling her to go but saying that she had a long day before her, or perhaps behind her, or both—and continued, as if Lou were twelve years old, to nag her about keeping her bedroom tidy or writing thank-you letters or washing her hair, in other ways she forced her on deplorably, so Lou herself thought. She tried to buy her too-sophisticated clothes, had given her a powder case for her birthday and attempted to discuss womanly things in which Lou

49

had no interest at all. She seemed worldly to her daughter and these hay-wire moral values were probably conventions anyhow. What will people think? She seldom went to church—Dorothea's funeral was the last time and someone's wedding would probably be the next. Religion was something that seemed to have no place in her life and gave no evidence of ever cropping up in her thoughts. Lou suspected that it sometimes cropped up in Dermot's, and made him feel uneasy and rather thirsty. She wondered if at those times he was anxious—as a lapsed Roman Catholic surely must be—about hell's fire. Young Father Blizzard was sure that this was so.

It was to the religion that Dermot had rejected, that Father Blizzard felt himself more and more forcibly drawn.

How much further he had been drawn since last she saw him, Lou was now anxious to find out. Yesterday she had bicycled once or twice past his lodgings and seen no one but his landlady standing back in the room, screened by a row of giant geraniums, and watching the road.

This morning Lou thought she might be lucky. She might meet Father Blizzard on his way back from the church school where he gave Scripture lessons. The rest of her unpacking could be left, but she straightened the bed-clothes and covered the bed—no hospital corners here. Then she hid her diary and went downstairs. Although she was going to meet her love, she had not even bothered to comb her hair.

. . . . .

As Tom crossed the factory yard, he knew that his grandfather was standing in the window of the office tower, as if upon the walls of Troy, watching the scene below. At any moment, his secretary's voice might come over the loudspeaker. 'Will Mr Wedgewood please report to Sir Alfred's office.' Only Tom, as he turned smartly about to obey the order, would recognise the venom in the young woman's voice. Once, mistakenly, he had taken her out to dinner and the usual drive to an isolated place afterwards. For some weeks there had been an encouraging warmth in her greeting, but then disappointment had chilled it. Now, she seemed not to notice him at all, was always frowning over papers or typing with great exertion when he went through the outer office. All the same, there would often be a smell of fresh face-powder in the air.

The yard was full of girls and women in green overalls, hurrying towards the canteen. This midday hazard was one of Tom's daily embarrassments.

'Isn't he sweet?' the girls asked one another as they passed him.

'He's a real dream boy. He reminds me of someone. Who does he remind *you* of?'

As they made their suggestions, he glanced once or twice at his watch and then took an old envelope from his pocket and studied it, as if it were something of considerable importance.

'You can see he isn't interested in us. I wonder who the letter's from. No, honest, he really is sweet. You can't say he isn't.'

They knew that in the factory he was nobody and could not retaliate. One day he might be able to, but by then they would all have left to get married, or those who were married already would have paid off the instalments on the television and could stay home and look at it.

They had reached the bicycle-racks and the remarks had become more bold, when Miss Parfitt's voice came over the loudspeaker. 'Will Mr Wedgewood come to Sir Alfred's office at once, please.'

'There, what a shame, he's got to go.'

'I shall miss him, won't you? What about his dinner?'

Burning with anger, Tom turned and began to go back across the road, walking, in spite of himself, more quickly.

'That's right, dear. Don't keep his lordship waiting,' one of the women shouted over her shoulder and some latecomers now hurrying past him laughed.

Up in his high office, built like a control tower above the works, Sir Alfred at the window was pleased to see that his grandson had quickened his pace, though he would rather have seen him running. The personnel manager always ran.

'Come over here, lad, and take a look,' he said as soon as Tom opened the door.

How he loved that window, Tom thought. He went over and stood beside the old man and suffered the weight of his arm on his shoulder. Any of those men crossing the yard below could have been jerked to attention and sent scurrying in another direction, as Tom himself had been, by a word from Miss Parfitt on the loud-speaker. At this distance Sir Alfred could deploy them as if they were toy soldiers.

'Now you want to watch those fellows unloading that van over there and tell me if you can't see a better way of doing it,' he said.

Tom looked sulky, only wishing to shrug off the hand resting on his shoulder.

'Well, you can't say there's nothing wrong, can you?'

'I suppose you mean Bert dropping that box,' Tom said.

'An occasional accident's neither here nor there, hasn't any im-portance. That's all estimated for in advance. If you're ever to make anything of this place after I've gone, you'll have to learn to ignore trivialities like that. Think on a larger scale. I've always done that—even when I hadn't two halfpennies to rub together —otherwise I'd have gone bust. No, lad, what matters is the basic pattern of work, and that's what you've got to look for. Or you'll get nowhere.'

Tom thought, 'He called me up here because he had an over-whelming urge to listen to his own voice and couldn't very well talk to himself, with Miss Parfitt out there listening.' Bert, perhaps flustered by the knowledge that he was being watched, now dropped another box.

'There, the basic pattern's all at fault,' said Sir Alfred. 'I'll tell you what, boy.'

He had not, of course, expected Tom to see it.

'One of them should stay at the tailboard to sort the goods. As it is they're all in one another's way, unpacking too slowly, carrying far too little at a time, colliding with one another as they turn. At a rough guess, I should say that they could nearly halve their time.

And time is money.' The last phrase had a ringing tone, as if it were freshly coined. 'There's a proper way of doing everything and that's the most economical way. Even I'm not too old to learn. A different unloading system must be worked out, to apply to the whole factory. That's more important than Bert dropping a box here and there. You were late this morning, boy.' He turned from the window and looked at Tom. 'How did that happen?'

'I couldn't get the car to start.'

'Again? I suggest that you take it for granted now that it won't start and get up half an hour earlier, to allow for it.'

'Yes, sir, I'll do that.'

Sir Alfred frowned. The boy sounded too negligently acquiescent, as if he did not mind what he promised as long as he could get away. He also disliked being called 'Sir' so much and would have preferred to be called 'Grandad' or something with a family sound to it.

'One other little thing. I noticed as you came through the office that you ignored Miss Parfitt. I didn't hear you say "Good morning". I've always looked upon every single person who's worked for me as having the right to be respected, and treated with courtesy. They may be my employees, but they're my fellow-beings too, and as such entitled to the civility of a "good morning" when we meet. And your education, your privilege, make it more incumbent, not less.'

That education, Tom thought sourly. His grandfather could never leave it alone. He must be thinking of it continually, with both envy and scorn. He exaggerated his early poverty to make his success more creditable.

'I don't think Miss Parfitt likes me much,' Tom said.

'It is not Miss Parfitt's place to have an opinion of you at all. Her likes and dislikes are beside the point.'

By now, Tom would have missed his lunch in the canteen, and although he was glad enough to escape the humiliations of the place, he was more hungry than cowardly.

'Miss Parfitt,' said Sir Alfred, taking up the telephone on his desk. 'Will you have the car sent round and ring up The Chequers to say that I shall be there in ten minutes—a table for two.'

'He reads my mind,' Tom thought. 'I'll have potted shrimps, roast duck, apple sauce, peas, no not peas, cauliflower, treacle tart, perhaps a vanilla ice-cream with it. And I'll be back at work at least half an hour late, thank God. It's all right when it suits him.'

'We can continue our chat over lunch,' his grandfather said. 'When we get back remind me to speak to Bert about dropping goods.'

He took off his heavy black-rimmed spectacles, folded them carefully, wrapped them in a piece of chamois leather and put them into their case. He was absorbed as he did so and had an air of reverence, for he looked after his possessions as if they were sacred objects, and nothing irritated him more than to see Tom scraping his car-wing on a gatepost or leaving things lying about—a habit of infuriating negligence he had from his mother, who never locked any doors, let the sun fade the carpets and had lost her engagement ring when planting some bulbs. 'It was insured,' she had said.

Tom, seated beside his grandfather in the hearse-like motor, was ignored by his workmates in the yard; they seemed not to have seen him pass. He had the worst of both worlds here, where it was hard work to make friends and he was suspect and stripped of independence. 'I'll tell him what he can do with his job,' the other men would say. Dermot would have said it too; but Tom sullenly and silently held on and felt that he lowered his self-esteem by doing so.

The gatekeeper saluted as the car turned into the road. Tom was looking in the other direction, but his grandfather lifted his cigar, in acknowledgment. Outside the factory gates it was another world and Tom leaned back against the pearl-grey upholstery in the too-hot car and closed his eyes. Why, he wondered, did he hang on so doggedly, scrambling in late day after day, wishing the hours away. He had no ambition to rule that world, to stand up in the office window, watching. He was terrified of making snap decisions and had no luck with them. He would go bankrupt, no doubt. From clogs and back to clogs in three generations was a brutish phrase he thought they used in the north.

When he opened his eyes again, the car was being slowed up by traffic. A flag flying on the bonnet was called for, he decided, and, while he was at it, added a few outriders on motor-bicycles.

Sitting behind the chauffeur, his grandfather held on to a tasselled cord and tapped his knee gently with the other hand. Tom examined with immense distaste the white fingers and the yellowing ribbed nails, like horrible old sea-shells with all lustre salt-scoured from them. Torturing himself, he noted the great stomach buttoned tightly into dark trousers and draped with a watch-chain. Without lifting his eyes he could complete the picture—the hooked nose, the aggressive black eyebrows and, especially, those even false teeth, as white as china, and the liver-coloured spots scattered over his cheeks. Any sort of old age disgusted him and this most of all. He was stifled in the slow-moving car, shut in with the old man, who for years had never gone out in the rain, for fear of getting bronchitis—or stepped a yard from his front door without putting on a hat. To think of him sitting down on the grass was absurd. As if sickened by the idea of decay, Tom's thoughts suddenly swarmed towards the evening, when he could be free and take some cold air into his lungs. He would drive fast in his open car and drink a great deal and eat indigestible things and, when he had courted all dangers and ailments, would entice Ignazia into some damp undergrowth and there make love to her, which, as well as asking for rheumatism, would be immoral, too.

. . . . .

Father Blizzard had almost ridden past Louisa—he was so short-sighted; but just in time he saw her and put on the brakes. She stood, hesitating and blushing, under the budding lime-trees by the churchyard wall, where she had been standing for half an hour.

'Louisa! How nice!' he said.

('Louisa! How nice!' she would murmur to herself in bed that night, trying over and over again to remember exactly the musical, slightly catarrhal quality of the voice.)

'You are the very one who could help me this morning,' he said. 'If you are not too busy, that is.'

'No, I am not busy in the least.'

'Then will you come and help me to buy a birthday present for my sister? You could put yourself in her place better than I.'

He walked beside her, back to his lodgings, pushing his bicycle along in the gutter, rather bowed over it as it was a racing bicycle. The Vicar thought it unsuitable and wondered if a great many other things about his Curate were not unsuitable too.

The shopping would have to be done in the town, Father Blizzard explained. He had already had everything out in the village shop and found only dull handkerchiefs or head scarves printed with chianti bottles. They could go on the bus and have coffee in the Tudor tea-rooms. There was a funeral at two. Old Mrs Hall, he said, and he looked for a moment serious, touched by a slight sadness which moved Lou deeply.

He propped his bicycle against the wall at the side entrance to his lodgings, stooped and pulled off the trouser clips from his ankles and tried to shake out the creases. Lou knew that this performance Tom would have thought boyish and absurd, and her love made her indignant with her knowledge. It was a disloyalty and she tried to abandon it.

When they were sitting together in the bus, she felt completely happy, without knowing that to feel so is such a rare experience that it might never come to her again. The very knowledge would have made something else of it. This morning was something she recognised as having been waited for, but with wavering degrees of hope. As the miracle had come about, she simply accepted it, but was taking it in little sips, blissfully restrained: for instance, she had not yet raised her eyes to look at his face.

The small cloud that had hovered while he was taking off the bicycle clips had quite dissolved. She said very little and looked out of the bus window as they descended the hill between beech-trees. She saw one of her friends, riding off to a gymkhana—that was obvious from the beautifully plaited horse's tail. The friend—as the bus passed—raised her crop, and Lou lifted her hand and smiled through the dusty window, feeling like the Queen going to open Parliament.

It was pleasant to know that the morning was not nearly half over yet. She had no plans about it in her mind, no expectations that might remain unsatisfied; really nothing could possibly happen to cause disappointment, and it was for this reason especially that the experience was rare and might never recur.

The shopping induced gaiety and intimacy, a holiday—almost honeymoon—mood took them, in which everything, everyone, seemed perfectly lunatic and incongruous. Father Blizzard was reminded of sunny mornings abroad, expeditions into villages to buy something for the sake of buying, choosing picture postcards with such care, writing them at a café table, going back to buy stamps and then seeing at the back of a shop window some object or other too preposterous, too absurd, to be missed. This morning, with Lou, he felt the same light-heartedness, for hers was contagious.

Lou's morning—though unthreatened by disappointments—was to have one or two moments of being clouded by anxiety; for instance, about the tray of bracelets at the jeweller's. When he asked her to choose one from them for his sister's present, she wanted him to know that she herself would never have worn the ones with charms hanging from them; but unfortunately they were the cheapest. Smoothing the wide strip of fine chain she so much preferred, she was wondering if he could afford it and how she could give any opinion that would not embarrass him. Curates are always poor, she thought, and she put down the best bracelet and sorted dubiously among the others. As soon as she had put it aside, he picked it up and said, 'I can read your thoughts, you know,' and she smiled with relief as if the present were for her, and was still relaxed with pleasure when they sat down at one of the tipsy little tables in the Tudor tea-rooms. One hazard was dealt with, she felt.

Then a worse one threatened. Father Blizzard took off his spectacles and began to polish them, very slowly and carefully, on his handkerchief. While he was doing this, he glanced round the room as if interested to see what he made of it with his unaided vision. He seemed quite unconscious of his appearance, of the bare, defenceless look he had without the glasses, of the furiously red mark across the bridge of his nose. At the sight of his weak, lustrous, naked eyes, Lou began to panic. He had become a stranger to her and she was terrified of pitying him. Her sense of disloyalty was insufferable and she bent her head and tried to engage the attention of a little cat which was walking between the tables; but the cat would not be made use of. Flicking her fingers at him, trying to entice with a piece of biscuit, she struggled to find something ordinary to say.

Her mother's and Tom's attitude to Father Blizzard was probably a reflection of their attitude to religion; Tom was briefly derisive and permanently impatient and Kate was indifferent. The last attitude was the more poisoning in its effect.

'You look worried,' said Father Blizzard, for she had given up trying to attract the cat and now was frowning as she spooned some skin off her coffee.

He had not said it in a teasing way, but seriously, and as if she were his own age.

'Our house is hell,' she said, deciding not to quibble about her difficulties or to tone them down in any way.

'It's one phrase in Shakespeare that never sounds freshly minted,' he said. 'It must have been said so many thousands of times both before and since.'

She was glad that he had finished polishing his spectacles and had put them on again.

'I was exaggerating,' she admitted, for she had not known that she was quoting something from Shakespeare and the fact laid too much stress upon her words. 'I meant that we are all at sixes and sevens. When Father was alive everything went more smoothly, and I'm sure that I'm not just remembering all the best parts as one does about one's youth. I used never to think about them—Mother and Father—I don't think one *should* have to think about one's parents. Now, I never stop thinking about Mother and wondering what she's going to get up to next. It won't be for my good whatever it is.'

'At her time of life,' he began, and the most alarming blush came out across her forehead. 'Oh, heavens, he is going to talk about sex,' she thought, trying to arm herself with composure.

He broke a biscuit, considered the two halves, popped one piece into his mouth and frowned. Then he said: 'Tom's grown up, his interests can't really be there, at home, any longer. Your mother must know that one day, not so far away, you'll want to leave her, too. She has to keep things as they are, and both of you in her thoughts and arrangements, but know that you might fly off and leave her at any moment. *She* won't decide when that will be, and she goes on caring for you both and trying at the same time to be ready for her life to become suddenly empty.'

The blush had receded. Lou even felt a little let down.

'She can't ever be alone now that she's got Dermot,' she said. 'He's there all day.'

'He may help her to get over the loneliness, but I don't suppose he will understand it. My mother, who is very close to me, has told me of the sense of deprivation women feel when their job of bringing up children comes to an end and there is no more for them to do.'

'She shouldn't fuss him with her troubles,' Lou thought, with a sudden gust of annoyance. She felt coldly towards the woman she imagined as, for some reason, very much older than Kate, white-haired, dismal, weeping into her son's handkerchief while he stood awkwardly by. 'I expect she revels in it,' she thought, and she looked with hostility at the trolley of home-made cakes the waitress was pushing by the table, and then she gave a glance round the café at the talkative women with their shopping baskets. 'I'll never grow up like them,' she thought.

'You shouldn't worry about your mother,' Father Blizzard was saying. 'Though it is very nice of you.'

'Everything has changed so, that's the trouble—Tom's very cagey. He leads a secret life and just comes in for meals. I think my mother gets jealous, and that's why she married Dermot; perhaps she thought that she would be getting someone quite young; who would be a bit like a son, but who would have to take her everywhere with him.'

'Are you sure that you think that? It would be better if you didn't. I think she married for love, as most people do.'

'Yes, I expect so, but there may have been motives she didn't understand.' Lou sounded sophisticated enough. She licked the top of her finger and pressed it into some candied sugar that had fallen off her bun. 'As a matter of fact, I think they were in love even before Father died. She always seemed excited and laughed a lot when Dermot came to the house, which he didn't very often, as I'm sure my father disliked him, and who could blame him, if he did? Oh, there's been trouble with Mother for years—Father's illness, when she looked so pinched-up and miserable, and we couldn't comfort her. We were terrified ourselves, anyhow! And then when he died. I know it was so much worse for her, though I felt my own heart was broken for ever and ever. But in no time at all she married Dermot—actually, we could see that coming a mile off—Tom and I. And now she's so different, such a very different person, much too gay for her age one minute, and over-tired and irritable the next; drinks too much, I should think, can't be bothered with her old friends—and after all, they're *my* friends' parents, most of them, and I've got to live in the place. I was left out of the Dixons' dance last holidays, and I'm sure it was because Mother hadn't asked them back for such ages.'

Now he did smile and she pulled herself up, realising that she had been sullen and aggrieved.

'I hope you don't think I'm disloyal,' she said. 'Of course, I suppose I am; but to *you*, surely . . .'

'We must pray for her,' he said simply.

'She would laugh if she heard you saying that.'

'It wouldn't matter.'

'She's condescending about my religion. "Nice time at church?" she asks when I get back—a sort of vague voice, not going to listen to the answer. I can tell.'

'Indifference is hard to bear.'

'I must tell you what happened once when I was young. I had a friend who suddenly became very religious. She made a beautiful little altar in her bedroom, with candles and so on. I was mad to have one like it and when I asked Mother if I could, she said, "Yes, darling, if you promise to clear it up afterwards." I felt so hurt about it at the time, but I suppose I see the funny side of it now. "Yes, darling, if you clear it up afterwards." Can you believe a mother would be so off-hand and cynical? I was too proud to have the altar after that but I didn't discard my religion, like some game I was bored with, though I know that she expected it of me. It was the same thing again last year when I was confirmed. "Of course, darling, you know I'd love to come." And so she did, and made me feel self-conscious. And she came the next Sunday to Communion, too, and went up to receive, if you please, after all those years and years of never bothering, and not believing. I knelt beside her and tried to put the word "hypocrisy" out of my mind.'

Father Blizzard was conscious of two people at the next table having fallen silent, although they were smiling at one another.

'Some more coffee?' he asked Lou, in a very low murmur he hoped she would copy.

Quickly comprehending, she shook her head and looked confused, but when he smiled, her face brightened with amusement. She gazed confidently back at him, so candid and trusting. Well, here I am, she seemed to say.

He was touched by the look she gave him and thought that she must be at the brink of losing that expression for ever, and, as if she sensed that she had moved him too much, she leaned forward and said in her most schoolgirlish voice: 'As a matter of fact, it was Valerie Dixon who had the altar. And she's the one whose dance I didn't get asked to.'

He looked at his watch and beckoned the waitress. 'We must talk again,' he said.

'Oh, yes.'

'Though, I'm afraid I'm rather tied up for a day or two,' he added, dashing her hopes of another chat the very next morning. 'It's my week for the cemetery, you see.'

. . . . .

Dermot wondered why he had not gone right into the shed and made quite sure that the white glimmer in the darkness was a piece of flint or chalk. Instead, he had shut the door, and stepped back into the sun. If the place had been carpeted with mushrooms, it could hardly have made much difference to him.

He strolled down the garden away from the house. He looked sullen and was thinking about his mother. In his pocket, his hand touched the envelope containing the bill for Kate's Christmas present. Because of that and other similar anxieties he knew that he must make one of his hated excursions to London. He would take his mother out to lunch, to some cheap place, pretending that he had heard it was amusing. 'Great fun,' he would keep saying as they sat perched on high stools in a coffee bar, eating pieces of decorated rye bread. He would allow—even encourage—her to speak of jobs she thought she could pull strings for. 'Shall we stroll back to the flat?' he would ask her, unless it were raining really torrentially. 'Strolling', he was sure, sounded as if it might be done for pleasure; it had a leisurely sound and suggested fine weather even if there wasn't any. 'Walking' had a hint in it of expediency and economy. At the flat, just before leaving and when the job was almost settled (except for a final word from Edwina to whoever it was that mattered), he would suddenly say, and make it seem as if he had almost let it slip his mind, 'Could there just be the slightest loan on *account* of the job, do you think? As I'm in London, I must get something for Kate.' Tiding over, he called it. 'Could you tide me over for a while, Mother dear?' Sometimes she made it easy for him, glossing over the occasion with laughing remonstrances. At other times, she exacted her toll with questions she wanted answered, not always about the matter in hand, for she would use the opportuι ity to try to assuage old curiosities.

'What a morning!' Mrs Meacock shouted to him. He had not seen her come from the back of the house, and wished that she had not seen him, standing as he was, stock-still, gazing at a piece of paper. She would think he had come into the garden to read it secretly and would imagine a love-letter, or even what it really was. Putting it back into his pocket, he made his way round the bushes towards her. She had lifted a cloche and was picking some parsley.

'It makes one think of holidays,' she said.

For twenty years, she had saved her money to go on a cruise. It was over now, but her constant reference to it was not.

'How you and Madam would love Bermuda,' she said. 'I can just picture you there. It just is Paradise on earth.'

She smiled, looking round at the muddy, leaf-strewn garden, as if it had been changed into a hot, white beach. Every day, the visions grew more beautiful in her memory.

'I could always hold the fort here,' she said, suddenly letting the vision go, for there were savoury things to be made, and puddings to whip up. She put the cloche back over the parsley—it was not Bermuda after all and there might be a frost to come—and went back to the house. Dermot had said nothing.

'He's not himself,' thought Mrs Meacock, for, under that roof and elsewhere, too, they were watching for the marriage to disintegrate. Conscious of this, Dermot became self-conscious. The same awkward surveillance from his mother had made him, as a boy, uncertain how to behave. When he had shown off, he had been humbled; the sulkiness he was so much blamed for was only a baffled retreat from his own mistakes. By the time he reached school, he was already settled into the habit of never being himself, deliberately displaying one inadequacy to mask another, trying to hide the real fault, not necessarily the worst. In defeat, his high spirits exceeded what courage demanded, and was called heartlessness. In love affairs, he knew he had been truly restless, and he stood now staring down at the row of cloches, thinking about love. He had never doubted its existence, only feared his own incapacity. He remembered how he had extricated himself from each affair, struggling to conceal how little he had cared, covering his retreat with bouquets of flowers, and only recently had wondered if they had seemed wreaths for a graveyard to the women who received them. If he had been loved, he had not really known it. He had tried to save their faces, seeing the situation from his own requirements.

At the moment, face-saving appeared a trivial thing—an insult to love, as he now experienced it. He turned and walked slowly towards the house. Ethel, also watching him, caught his eye and flapped a duster out of the window and withdrew.

Kate, not his mother, must help him, Dermot decided. Money's only money, he told himself. It's only for spending, and I spent it. All it has to do with love, is to provide a booby trap.

He looked for Kate, but could not find her, and it was nearly one o'clock before she came back, and then she looked sad and preoccupied.

She had been to look at Dorothea's house, as she still thought of it, had fetched the key from a woman who at times went in to light fires and open windows. Disconsolately she had walked about the stuffy rooms, where light slanting through venetian blinds striped the sheeted furniture.

After the funeral, Araminta had soon been sent away to France; later, Charles, her father, had gone abroad too—though for some reason, perhaps because he went on business, it was referred to as 'overseas'. Since then, although she had vaguely promised to, Kate had not brought herself to enter the house. She remembered too painfully the last time when she had helped Araminta to serve tea to her relations—that poor, stunned girl, moving from one to the other with frozen courtesy. Kate had never imagined them living there again. They would make other plans, she thought. The house would be put up for sale.

This morning, wondering what could be done to make it less dreadful for father and daughter when they returned, she had lifted the dust covers and tried to silence a dripping tap. The drawing-room smelt sooty and some newspaper in the grate was black.

They were making a mistake in coming back, she decided, drawing a line with her finger on a dusty sill. The house, like Dorothea, could never be revived. Kate locked up and returned the key.

'I wondered where you'd gone,' Dermot said.

He was aggrieved that, just when he had wanted her most, had suddenly hurried indoors to take her into his arms and tell the truth for once and find refuge in her, she had disappeared, and no one knew where, and had returned now in this abstracted mood.

'I went down to Dorothea's—to the Thorntons',' she said. 'I thought there might be things to see to before they come back.'

'And were there?'

By half past twelve his resolution had failed. Now he felt antagonistic and, pouring out a second drink, thought that he would do anything to keep the truth from her.

'A chimney to be swept, a tap needing a washer,' she said, knowing that he was not interested and was asking questions for the sake of talking, not listening. 'They are making a great mistake in coming back, I am sure.'

'You will be glad, with your plans for Tom and that girl.'

'I haven't any plans; you know that. And what would it matter if I had? Oh, yes, of course, I shall be glad to see her.'

'Not Charles?'

Without knowing, she had stressed her last word, and Dermot had noticed it.

'There's Lou at the gate, with the Curate, Father What's-his-name,' she said.

Dermot came to the window where she was.

'They're an unlikely couple,' he said.

'I *don't* want Charles to come back,' she thought. He would expect her to have stayed the same, and she had not. People must change when different things happen to them, she told herself, and felt annoyance with her old friend, as if he had already voiced a complaint.

Father Blizzard was moving on.

'He is giving her quite a roguish smile,' said Dermot.

'You can't possibly see from here.'

'I have eyes like an eagle. By the way, one good thing this morning—the mushrooms have begun. I was thinking they never would.'

'Oh, how exciting.'

'Yes, I must be sure to tell everyone not to open that door. Goodness gracious, he patted her head. *Should* she be walking out with him like this? Oh, dear, she ought to know better than to stand there staring after him.'

'Don't tease her, Dermot.'

'You ought to know that I never would. That's right, dear girl, you come along in. He must have looked back. She's waving.'

'Everyone watches *me*,' he thought. 'I'll do *my* share.'

Lou had closed the gate and light as a leaf came dancing up the path.

. . . . .

At half past five, the factory gates were opened, and a policeman on point duty tried to untangle the traffic. In the swarm of bicycles, even Sir Alfred's car was held up. He stared irritably before him, like a wasp caught in a spider's web, impatient that he, for all his power, could not escape. His chauffeur blew softly but constantly on the horn, making slow progress through swerving and colliding bicycles. Nevertheless, Sir Alfred would not for anything have set out five minutes earlier to ease the congestion. He preferred to leave and be seen leaving at the same time as his men. There seemed some virtue in this to him, and he would not have believed that other people saw the thing differently. 'I've never asked a man to do what I wouldn't do myself, or haven't done,' he liked to say. This was untrue as well as uninteresting.

Tom waited for the rush to be over, and watched his grandfather's car, finally extricated, pressing on up the hill to the hideous plum-coloured turreted house which smelt like its owner—of cigar smoke and camphor—and where he had lived in great loneliness since his wife had died.

Ignazia was waiting by the traffic lights. She was wearing red woollen stockings and a raincoat. Her hair, this evening, was piled up high and held there with a comb. Tom, driving up to the kerb and leaning over to open the door for her—he had no manners, Dermot said—was a little cast down at seeing this particular hairstyle, for it went usually with her most dominating, scornful mood. He would rather see it loose—a sign that she was feeling gay and compliant.

Firstly, she began, he was late. She had been standing for five minutes, exposed to several objectionable remarks from men passing by. 'Those stockings, you see,' Tom said. 'Shall we go to the cinema?' Secondly, she had a headache.

So he would have to take her to some expensive Thames-side pub and in this grand, headmistressy mood she would be sure to order smoked salmon.

This happened. 'Well, I can pay,' Tom thought, 'but when I have I'll be skinned.' He was depressed and disappointed. Even apart from money matters, he preferred Ignazia in her loose-haired, cinema, fish-and-chips, love-in-the-back-seat mood; and that was the mood he had visualised for tonight, to offset the frustrations he had suffered all day. As it was, she was only underlining the frustrations, especially, of course, the financial ones. For the hundredth time, he thought how little it would mean to his grandfather to ease him, Tom, of those particular worries, and he wondered if it was from envy of youth that old people kept what they had—even if it were a great deal—and then pretended that their meanness was in the interests of the deprived. Not only the really elderly either, Tom thought. The middle-aged—his mother, for instance—could save him from many anxious contrivances, spoilt evenings, gaieties forsworn, simply for the price of what she paid for a hat. What she had squandered on the Boudin in the drawing-room—a drab little picture, no more than eight inches by five—was a particular grievance. It pointed to how much she had to squander. 'And Dermot does all right,' he thought.

Ignazia, who had her own grievances, began to go over them. Her employers had a wonderful excuse for parsimony. They sheltered behind the law, refusing to pay her a penny more than the small amount that as an alien domestic help she was allowed to earn. Her clothes were wearing out, a laddered stocking was a tragedy and she suffered it as such.

'They must have spent fifty pounds on the cocktail party,' she told Tom, 'and it was all over in two hours. At half past eight, everyone had gone away. I don't blame them. No one could have liked it. It was not very gay. I had to carry round some canapés and people stretched right across the tray to pick out the ones with cod's roe on them. They thought it was caviare. Even when they had eaten it, some still thought it was. When that was gone, they lost interest. I was walking round with the tray for the rest of the time, asking people, but they would not change their minds. Some women stared crossly at me. The men pinched me. But so much money wasted,' she said, returning to the theme, for Tom was never roused by the insults she suffered.

At the next table, there was some competitive discussion about champagne, between two men dining together. 'I always prefer the Bollinger to the Moët,' said the one who seemed to be the host. He thoughtfully sipped and swilled the wine round his mouth. 'It's got more of a nip in it,' he added, when at last he had wrenched it down his throat. His companion solemnly agreed, but put in a word or two for Krug. Tom winked at Ignazia, who shrugged.

The room was half-empty, candle-lit. Close to the windows, the weir tumbled and thundered—a romantic background, but too muffled to cover conversation. 'Dermot Heron,' Tom suddenly heard from the next table.

'Yes, of course. Saw him not long ago at Aintree, funnily enough. He was fairly high at the time.'

'I never saw him when he wasn't.'

The men, celebrating some business deal perhaps, sipped their wine thoughtfully and sometimes took sole bones out of their mouths.

'Saw him once in The George with his wife.'

'Wife? My God, I'd have laid any odds he'd never marry. I hope she's got plenty of money, that's all. Who is she?'

'My mother,' Tom said loudly, without looking up from his plate. Ignazia hardly stirred, watching the men's faces with very little interest.

'It hadn't occurred to me I had addressed you.' Much put out, the man decided to attack.

'It's perfectly true, you didn't.'

Tom took up the pepper-mill and turned it once or twice over his smoked salmon. It was a more authoritative gesture than fiddling with wine-glasses, as the other two were doing.

'Times have certainly changed,' one of them said. 'In my young day, listening to other people's conversations was a bit off, we always considered.'

'So you didn't enjoy the party?' Tom asked Ignazia, who shrugged again.

'The height of rudeness,' Tom overheard as he lovingly ate his smoked salmon. He could not have sat and watched Ignazia eating hers while he saved a shilling or two drinking lentil soup himself. Such subterfuges degraded him, he thought.

'You didn't want champagne, did you?' he asked Ignazia, who for once looked rather startled. 'I always think it's a drink for one's elevenses.'

This odd word Ignazia did not know and when he had explained it, Tom glanced at the other table. The conversation from that direction was intermittent now, and the voices low. They had all behaved ridiculously, he suddenly thought. And whose fault was it, but his mother's?

'I like your smoked salmon,' said Ignazia.

For a minute, he thought that she was coolly asking for the rest of his, and then he realised that she was only being condescending about English food.

'That's very gratifying.'

In public places, they behaved challengingly to one another, involved in rather a tiring competitiveness; for Tom could not be serious except under cover of darkness, and then about only one thing, and Ignazia—for her part—felt she had much to combat in the life about her. The self-satisfaction of the English she would not indulge, and their indifference as to whether she did so or not was exasperating.

'Two Rognons au Madère,' said the host at the next table.

'Rognons au Madère for two,' the waiter said, pompously correcting his pronunciation.

'What about some mushrooms with it?' the host asked his guest, who seemed to judge the matter carefully, and then nodded.

'Extra mushrooms, sir?' the waiter asked in a dubious, reproving voice. 'There are, of course, mushrooms in the dish itself.'

'It will be very nice here in the summer,' said Ignazia. 'We can sit by the window and look at the river.' She drew back a curtain and put her forehead close to the pane, but it was quite dark outside, and she could see nothing. The sound of the weir seemed to increase in volume whenever she thought of it. As she shifted her thoughts, it became a soft confusion in the background.

'It seems so close, as if the water is running underneath this very room,' she said.

'I've seen it running *through* the room,' said Tom, 'and swans swimming in one door and out of another. There are often floods round here.' He explained a flood.

'I should like to see this,' she said wistfully. Next winter where would she be, she wondered. She could foresee the succession of rainy days, the low clouds crowding overhead, and the alarming fog. Before that, the summer days with colourless skies and very often something called drizzle, which was as disheartening as its name. If she married Tom, she would be imprisoned here because of his work—somewhere in the Thames Valley for the rest of her life, perhaps perched up on the surrounding chalk hills under the wet beech-trees, or by the river itself, with the swans swimming in and out of their drawing-room every winter. They could have holidays in Spain, but not for more than three weeks of a year—enough to unsettle her, or break her heart. She tried to come to her decision—as if Tom had really asked her to marry him.

At the next table, the two men looked suspiciously at their plates while they were being served. Then in silence each took a mouthful. They looked doubtfully at one another.

'Tough,' the host said, frowning.

The other nodded, as if he were sorry that he could not deny it. Bothered with gristle, he put his fork to his mouth.

Yet, thought Ignazia, if Tom were to go into the wine trade, there could very well be constant journeys to Spain. It might even be expedient for them to live there altogether. He had so often said how dreary and uncongenial he found the factory and his grandfather. She had once hinted to him of an influential cousin who had a connection with a firm of sherry exporters, and Tom had seemed tempted; he had wavered, she thought, and wore for a moment a look of pride and disdain as he designed his farewell to his grandfather. Unfortunately, the cousin was a very distant one, and his connection with the exporters turned out to be vague. She had written home to enquire. And also—she must always come back to it—Tom had not asked her to marry him. Judging all his countrymen by his behaviour, she thought how immoral Englishmen were, who took for granted that, after an evening, quite unromantic and perhaps full of sharp retorts and acts of negligence, girls who were almost strangers to them should soften suddenly and yield to love, with love not mentioned at the time, and marriage mentioned at no time.

Her thoughts had made her cheeks red with indignation, and

she looked crossly at the other Englishmen at the next table, with whom, for some reason, Tom appeared to be annoyed.

The waiter, taking up their plates, said with casual deference: 'Some Stilton, sir, or a slice of pineapple?'

Both men hesitated, having first glanced hopefully at a trolley full of bright trifles and quivering jellies.

'I'm going to have something off the trolley,' said the host. He tried to cover his feeling of unmanliness with robust defiance. His guest nodded with relief.

'Gâteau, I think,' he said, pointing to something smothered with chocolate and chopped nuts.

'Yes, gâteau will do fine,' said his friend.

They watched the large wedges being cut, but as soon as they put their forks to them, their playfulness vanished. They looked with quiet disappointment at the dull sponge that the chocolate had hidden.

'Years since I had anything like this,' said one. 'I haven't a very sweet tooth as a rule. I usually prefer cheese.'

'I usually do myself,' his friend agreed.

'Would you like some cheese?' Tom asked Ignazia.

'As you like,' she said mysteriously. 'Is it nice here on Saturdays? I find I can go out on Saturdays too.'

'We should never get a table,' Tom said.

'You could ask. I very much like the smoked salmon. It is wonderful English food. The kind I have liked best since I was here.'

'It isn't a particularly English food,' Tom said, thinking wistfully of fish and chips, which was. 'You could come and have supper with us at home.'

'Thank you.' She did not attempt to sound enthusiastic. Then she brightened a little, and said that the arrangement might not be convenient to his mother; but unfortunately it appeared that nothing pleased Kate more than for Tom and Louisa to bring their friends home at any time. That was once true, he reflected, remembering all the impromptu parties there had been, and the occasions when he had invited girls to the house and his mother had taken as much trouble as she had when she and his father were entertaining their own friends.

Lately, he felt some constraint when he asked Ignazia there. His mother's voice was gay and welcoming enough and perhaps Ignazia herself was unaware of any effort that was made; but effort was demanded, he knew, and under some difficulty was met, and Kate never quite managed to look at the girl. It was this that was wrong, he had realised after a time. His mother seemed self-conscious and was constantly busy, finding things to attend to, always turning aside or lowering her eyes.

He watched the two men leaving, saw the waiter's geniality switched off as soon as they had gone through the door.

'They spoilt my evening, and I spoilt theirs,' he thought.

'Saturday, then,' he said, and Ignazia nodded.

[3]

I WANTED to know, Mother, what all this is about Lord Auden?'
Dermot said.

Edwina found it delightful to say firmly: 'No, I won't discuss it,
my dear. Kate was very definite about the matter. In fact, a
touchier person than I might have felt that she was rude. However,
I understand her manner by now.'

'But it's my concern . . .'

'Exactly.'

'And you should have known that in the first place.'

'I did. But when do I ever see you to discuss anything? When
you are wanting to borrow money, Dermot.'

He wished that he had not given her time to answer her own
question. She had done it too promptly and, in doing so, rendered
his visit useless.

'Where did *that* come from?' he asked, glaring crossly at a
picture of Queen Victoria opening the Great Exhibition. It was
painted in black and sepia upon silk and hung opposite him above
the pale green chaise-longue on which his mother was sitting.

'It belongs to Lord Auden,' she said, and she spread out her
plump, mottled hands, palms downwards, and examined her
nails, as if her manicurist had just this minute finished them.

'I suppose her lips are pursed,' Dermot thought. When reading
the words, he had always imagined such an expression. A tightly
shut purse, too, he decided—auguring failure for him.

But a girlish sense of importance was too much for her, and she
glanced up at the picture and said: 'It's amusing, don't you think?'

'Hideous.'

'But amusingly hideous,' she insisted. 'People notice it and

74

laugh. They talk about it, and then say, "Where did you find it?" That's why it's hanging there. It gives me a chance to mention our little project. "You *must* find something ghastly for me, too," they say. Which reminds me, darling, if you should chance upon any old brass milk churns anywhere. They were before your time, of course, but you know what I mean. Or any Jubilee beer mugs. You might see those in a pub.'

'What do I do if I do? Make an offer?'

'No. Say absolutely nothing. Don't give a sign of having noticed them, but as soon as you can, get on the telephone to me. And, of course, those china barrels. But too many people are after them.'

'There are two in The Bird in Hand at home. One is pink and gilt and labelled "Bishop" and the other is green and called "Shrub". I've no idea what either means.' He had gazed at them for long enough at a time, wondering.

She leant forward and stared at him, her hands now clasped together. 'What sort of an inn is it?'

'Poky.'

'Has it been modernised?'

'They've put beer pipes up from the cellar now.'

'No, no. I mean—are they sophisticated people? What sort of décor is there?'

'Nothing very much. Just the ordinary pub stuff. Varnished pike over the door, a picture called "A Game of Whist!" ' He had stared at that for long periods, too.

Edwina got up and walked about the room. She had slipped her shoes off while sitting down and now tiptoed round in stockinged feet—tiptoeing and whispering, as if she might otherwise disturb the landlord of The Bird in Hand, and rouse his suspicions about the value of his barrels.

'He probably hasn't a clue,' she said. 'What are the handles like? You know, the things they draw the beer with?'

'China, with pansies painted on them.'

She nodded. 'They might be imitation,' she said.

'Imitation handles?'

She shook her head impatiently. 'I must go down there at once.'

Most places in the country were 'down' from London to her—even if considerably north.

'What a fool I am,' Dermot thought. To Edwina he said: 'If you're thinking of doing some shopping for Lord Auden at The Bird in Hand, I can assure you they're not the sort of people who would take kindly to the suggestion.'

'We can but try. You'll help me, darling. You know them, and you've your father's charm.'

'Why should you expect me to be interested? Just now, when I mentioned that I was, you refused to discuss it.'

'It was because of Kate. The last thing I want to do is to interfere or to come between you in any way. And she quite frightened me off, you know.'

'Kate can't stop me taking a job. I'm my own master.'

She shrugged. 'It's what I've always felt, but couldn't say. "He's his own master," I thought.' (The absurd phrase, Dermot noted—wondering why he had used it.) ' "She is silly to tie him to her apron strings. No man wants to kick his heels about the place all day!" '

'I'm bored,' he said. 'And I dare say the job would bore me even more. But when I think of the quantities of rubbish I've seen lying about the countryside and you say that people will pay money for it . . . Are those filthy old moustache cups any good?' he suddenly asked. 'And shaving mugs?'

She turned round, with the cigarette box in one hand, its lid in the other, and nodded eagerly. 'People grow plants in them,' she said.

'She's not all there,' he thought.

'You see, you've got the idea. You must come with me to the shop. He's found the very place—just off Sloane Street—with a bow-fronted window. You'd adore it.'

He leaned back and smiled. For some reason, she remembered one of her birthdays when he was a little boy. He had worn the same smile while he watched her unwrapping her present from him—an egg-rack he had made at school. She had glanced up and seen the pleasure and pride upon his face. 'We were very close in those days,' she thought now. He noticed tears in her eyes and felt that he could understand. 'We are poles apart,' he thought, 'but she was always concerned for me. The antagonism is my fault—I neglected her.'

'In all frankness, I want the money,' he explained. 'I can't keep—'

'No, of course,' she said quickly, unable to bear hearing him say whatever it was that he couldn't keep doing. 'I could help you at first.'

His lips parted. He thought she meant to help financially, but then she said: 'I think I have quite a flair for it—for guessing what everyone will be hunting for in a few months' time. I started that craze for tea-urns years ago and I don't remember anyone having a bamboo bed-head before me.'

'A what?' Dermot asked, feeling disappointed and goaded beyond bearing.

'A bamboo bed-head. I'm sure the shop will be a little gold mine. It's just a question of raising some capital to stock it. Then it should soon start booming. Kate must see that.'

'She never will,' Dermot thought. 'She has too much sense.'

'Shall I come down and try to talk to her again?' Edwina asked, willing to brave as much for all their sakes. 'It never seemed particularly important to me to stand on my dignity. I've never been proud and, as long as *you* don't think I'm interfering, I don't mind how she snubs me.'

'I feel it would come better from me,' he said. 'And at the right time,' he said to himself.

The words were ominous, he thought. They suggested that she had an occasion in mind.

'I must pay my visit to The Bird in Hand,' she added. 'We can just drop in and say we have run out of cigarettes.'

'One doesn't need an excuse for going into a pub.'

'I just want our approach to seem quite casual. Otherwise they'll suspect that we're dealers. I've done quite a lot of this sort of thing here and there in my time. I'm not coming to it as a complete novice. I've even had things offered to me, without having to make suggestions—just picked them up for a song and sometimes for free. Years ago, I remember, when your father was still alive, an old woman in a village shop gave me a terra cotta teapot and wouldn't take a penny for it. She said it was ugly.'

'And so it was, I remember it.'

'I grew ferns in it. Do you think Kate could put me up—just Saturday to Monday?' She quickly covered what Dermot had intended to be a pause. 'I won't say a word about you know what.'

She looked at her wrist-watch and began to cram her feet into her shoes. 'Ask her,' she said. 'Telephone tomorrow.'

'Where are you going?' he asked, as she picked up her handbag.

'To a dress show and the chairs aren't numbered or anything, and I don't want to be stuck at the back. I'd no idea the time had gone by . . . but I'm so happy about it all, and I know that Wilfred will be, too. He has always doted on you. I'll see him tomorrow and, meanwhile, just keep quiet and have your eyes open for anything interesting. The most unlikely place is where to look. If you're taking a taxi to the station, you can drop me off on the way.'

'I have no money for taxis,' he said. He was desperate lest she should run away from him before he could come to the point. 'Or for anything else,' he added.

She opened her handbag and began to finger the notes. About seven pounds, he guessed, his hopes sinking. He could not help feeling annoyed.

'I'll write a cheque in the taxi,' she said.

At once, he stood up, and she quickly straightened the cushion he had been leaning against.

'And you'll ask Kate and telephone tomorrow?' she said again as they went downstairs, and this time received an answer. 'Well, that will be lovely.'

She opened the door at the head of the basement stairs and shouted some instructions in French, which were incomprehensible to Dermot, then she hurried out of the front door and he followed her. Going down Brompton Road, she took out her cheque book and, resting it on her handbag, began to write. Dermot looked out of the window.

'By the way, what happened about the mushrooms?' she asked.

'Someone left the door open. I lost the lot,' he said.

. . . . .

The church jumble-sale had little to do with love—no more than Lou's hopes of seeing Father Blizzard perhaps at some point during the afternoon. For that reason, she had let herself be roped in—as Miss Buckley put it, vividly suggesting the almost panicky unwillingness Lou felt.

At the pricing committee in the village hall, she was dumb with embarrassment. It was as if she had found herself on new terms with the staff at school, exposed to their bonhomie, and forced to see them in a completely different light—all of them suddenly mad, jaunty and effusive—and expected to share in their jokes.

Her mother had never been a committee woman. Always so busy, other women kindly said. She had certainly had plenty to do. She and Dorothea had gone for long walks, in winter along the deserted towing-path at Marlow, in summer on the chalky hill-slopes. They had sat idly by the fire while afternoons darkened and their neighbours returned from meetings. The door flying open might be Tom or Araminta back from school. 'Hello, my pet,' they'd say, each clasping in turn the cold, bright creature from outdoors, then resuming their conversation.

'Your mother's such a busy woman always,' Lou was told several times during the afternoon.

'She made a sponge cake for us one year,' Miss Buckley said. 'I remember Mother bought it, and it was as light as a feather.'

It seemed to be all that Kate had ever done and had become an accusing sponge cake by now, so long after; for Mrs Buckley had been dead for some years.

Louisa's afternoon was eventful. Fastidious, though discreet, indignation was roused by the worn, discoloured corsets sent in by the village schoolmistress. 'Least said, soonest mended,' Miss Buckley murmured. She raised her eyebrows questioningly at the others and, seeming to receive their assent, dropped the sordid parcel into a waste paper basket.

Mrs Shotover from the Post Office said it was disgusting that they should be expected to handle such things. She meant to find as much fault as she could, for the afternoon had begun badly for her. She had only removed her cardigan for a moment, feeling one of her hot flushes coming over her, and, turning to look for it a minute or two later, had found it laid out on a stall, marked four-pence. She was therefore delighted to discover signs of moth in the Duchess's fur necklet, which was like a bunch of thin, dead animals.

'She wouldn't have sent it otherwise,' someone pointed out.

'They'll get into everything else. Come on, pussy. After them! Rats!' Mrs Shotover said, shaking the fur at the caretaker's cat, who merely walked more widely of them all, on its way to the kitchen. They had a little more fun at the Duchess's expense, glancing sometimes at Lou for her reactions. She was miserably conscious of being watched. How would she shape? they were all wondering. Would she become an asset to the village, and who was it she favoured—her mother or her father? Most of them had known her since she was a little girl, but this was her first appearance as a person on her own. She knew it and, drearily trying to sort out pairs from a heap of old shoes, smiled in what she hoped was an open, jolly way, although she was suffering so much from feeling herself superior to their jokes. They were all so childlike, she decided, so innocent, so countrified.

She had been given the worst job—as was wholly proper, she knew; but she wondered who in the world would buy such lamentable objects. She prayed that someone would, for she wanted to do very well when the sale began.

'Goodness me!' Miss Buckley might say—and in Father

Blizzard's hearing, perhaps—when Lou handed in her takings. 'We've never done anything like as well as that with shoes before.'

She suddenly heard his name spoken, and she took up an old sandal and examined it—more closely than she would have done if she had been conscious of the action. He was mentioned in connection with his landlady, who had sent in an object which was puzzling them all, but soon they went on to mention him on his own account.

'I heard the Vicar hauled him over the coals,' Mrs Shotover said in a low voice, much lower than the Vicar's could have been, for young Shotover, at the back door of the Vicarage with a registered parcel, seemed to have heard it all.

' "It's not a day we recognise," or words to that effect, he was saying.'

' "Feast"! That's how Father Blizzard spoke of it. "I didn't know we *had* feasts in the Church of England," I said.'

'*Father* Blizzard!' said the caretaker's wife, coming from the kitchen with a tray of crockery. 'I'm certainly not saying "Father" to a slip of a boy like that. "Mr" was always good enough for Mr Phillips,' she said, speaking of the previous Curate. 'And "Mr" it shall continue to be.'

'He was good to old Mrs Hall before she died,' said someone who was apparently of no account, but at whom Louisa glanced with gratitude.

'I think it's an egg-cup stand without the egg-cups.' The butcher's wife held up the puzzling electro-plated object, and was ignored.

'It's the Assumption of the Virgin Mary we don't recognise,' Miss Buckley said knowingly.

'I must remember that to tell him,' Louisa thought, but at once decided that she must not. She could do nothing for him, kneeling there on the dusty floor, trying not to feel squeamish about other people's horrid cast-offs—or nothing more than hide her reddened cheeks if she could. She was bound to keep silent, for to speak up for him would make a fool of him, she felt.

'I can't see him lasting,' Mrs Shotover said. 'I've no objection whatsoever to Roman Catholics—in their rightsome place, that is. But how High we go is surely for the Vicar to decide, not for a boy like that.'

'I've wondered lately,' Miss Buckley said, 'if the Vicar himself isn't going a little Higher than I'm prepared to follow.'

'The Patronal Festival, you mean?'

'Not only that.'

Mrs Shotover nodded. She took off her cardigan again, but this time kept it hanging loose on her shoulders.

'I once went into Westminster Cathedral,' Miss Buckley said. 'I didn't care for it. "I could no more pray there, than fly to the moon," I said to Mother.'

'I know what you mean,' Mrs Shotover said, fanning her face with her handkerchief. Then she narrowed her eyes in a warning way, having seen Father Blizzard in the porch.

An awkwardness fell over them, for no one knew exactly what note to strike now, how to receive the Curate, without seeming two-faced to the others. As he came into the hall, the butcher's wife, who was determined to identify the mystery object, said: 'No, I'm sure it's the stand to one of those collapsible butter coolers.'

This time they turned their attention almost gratefully to her.

'You are quite right,' said Father Blizzard. 'And I have been sent along with the missing parts. Hallo, Louisa,' he said, touching her head lightly as he passed by.

'Is there anything I can do to help?' he asked. 'Any menial task? Any trivial thing that even I could manage?'

Miss Buckley turned aside to let the others, but not Father Blizzard, see her Mona Lisa smile.

'If money for the mission were not involved, one would have to feel guilty at shifting all this rubbish round from place to place,' he said. He looked at the old clothes, the piles of ancient gramophone records and dusty books, and at Louisa kneeling humbly on the floor by the heap of boots. 'It is terrible to help its progress,' he added.

Their silence reminded him that he must appear to be belittling their work, so he spoke again of the missionary fund. 'And what is *this* magnificent object?' he asked, with an attempt at joviality.

'It is the pogo-stick my brother and I played with when we were children,' said Miss Buckley, who felt that she had sacrificed it. Her brother's having been killed in the war, as everybody knew, made an added embarrassment for Father Blizzard.

Louisa, so new to Church work, had never before seen him with his parishioners and felt their attitude most painfully. 'My heart bleeds,' she told herself. She put two black shoes together, then saw that one had a stitched toe-cap, the other had not.

'I think that's that,' Mrs Shotover said, glancing round the hall. 'Two o'clock tomorrow, everyone.' ('*Please*,' the butcher's wife added to herself, thinking that Mrs Shotover domineered.) 'I should put the rest of those into a clothes basket, Louisa. Mark them down. All one price. People can sort them out for themselves. Shoes never do any good, anyhow!'

'So many wounded feelings this afternoon,' Lou thought. 'And now mine.'

Feeling that her efforts had been wasted and were seen to have been, she fetched the basket and did as she was told.

'Disgusting old boots,' Father Blizzard whispered, bending down beside her to help fill the basket. 'Embittering old jumble-sales.'

At once, she felt gay, and enlivened by a sense of conspiracy.

'Good-bye all,' Miss Buckley called from the doorway. 'Good-bye, Father Blizzard.'

Although she disapproved of him, she felt a little excitement in addressing him in this way, and it was evident in her voice.

Louisa went to the kitchen and washed her hands with a lump of gritty, yellow soap. In a cracked piece of looking-glass over the sink, she studied her face with dissatisfaction—her hair was untidy, and one eye looked swollen and bloodshot. When she returned only the caretaker's wife was left, and Father Blizzard, who was kicking an empty carton down the hall towards a pile of rubbish.

83

He turned and joined Louisa and they went to the door together.

'Good-bye, Mr Blizzard,' the caretaker's wife called after him.

'I don't think I've heard you utter a word yet,' he told Louisa, as he wheeled his bicycle away from the railings. 'I didn't know you could keep anything up for so long—especially silence.'

'I find them all too frightening.'

'Yes—I do, too. In my case it's a well-founded fear, since I'm in hot water everywhere, it seems.'

He pushed his bicycle, walking beside her through the village.

'Are you going to turn into a great Church worker?' he enquired. 'Is this the beginning I have witnessed?'

'It seems to have so little to do with religion,' she complained. 'That stuffy hall and the catty women and, as you said, the disgusting old boots.'

She looked up through the budding branches at the sky, as if with relief, and took a long breath. He looked up, too—briefly for, in doing so, he knocked his ankle on the bicycle pedal, and cursed.

'Those people who say that they can pray just as well under God's blue sky, while they're out walking the dog, better than in church. It's always God's blue sky. Or the wide arch of Heaven.'

'Miss Buckley couldn't pray in Westminster Cathedral. She could as soon fly to the moon, she said.' Louisa immediately wished she had not said this, but it was too late.

'God likes Gothic best,' he said casually. 'When did this interesting conversation take place?'

'This afternoon.'

He was silent.

They had come to the end of the village, and to Louisa's gate.

'My heart's not at home in this place,' he said. 'Too much is wrong. But no matter. I hope you sell out of boots tomorrow and don't catch leprosy.'

He had jumped on to his bicycle and gone before she could reply.

'Where have you been, dear girl?' Dermot asked her, as she entered the house. He had just come back from seeing his mother in London, and was standing in the hall, sorting the afternoon letters.

'Getting a jumble-sale ready. I'm so filthy. I feel I'll never get clean again. The awful junk—everything years old and unwanted. You can't imagine.'

He looked at her with interest, remembering Edwina's new hobby.

.   .   .   .   .

Kate was in her bedroom, scrubbing her hands. She had spent the afternoon at Dorothea's house, dusting books. They were not so much damp as unaired, unread, neglected, clenched—some of them—upon lost letters, forgotten photographs, and dried flowers. From one had fluttered a home-made birthday card, which, long ago, Araminta must have drawn for her mother—twenty-nine candles were crowded on a lumpy cake, done in pale, shiny crayon.

'How was Edwina?' Kate asked, when Dermot came looking for her.

She was amused that he had made excuses for going to see his mother. 'I wonder if he really loves her?' she had thought, but she could not take the idea quite seriously. He was touchy about her, Kate realised, defensive. His fists seemed to be tightened in readiness, lest anyone should find her as absurd as he did, or speak of her as slightingly.

'I didn't see much of her,' he said. 'She was going out, thank goodness. But the truly terrible thing is that she wants to come for the week-end.'

'Whatever for?' Kate asked, then tried to disguise her consternation. 'She would be bored to tears.'

'She wants to buy some of those old china barrels. Like a fool, I told her there were some in The Bird in Hand.'

Kate smiled, slowly drying her hands. 'Ah, she is foraging for Lord Auden, no doubt,' she said. 'Perhaps she is going into his business instead of you. Just think of the treasures she could find in Ethel's room.'

He stood watching gloomily, as she went through one drawer, then another, looking for something. 'There was a place for everything and everything in its place when we were first married,' he remembered. The change since then interested, but did not affect him.

'I shall have to let her know one way or the other,' he said.

'Of course she must come. There's nothing happening this week-end, as far as I know. Only Ignazia to dinner on Saturday, I think Tom said.'

Dermot sat down on the window-seat and began to look through some books Kate had left there.

'They're mine,' Kate said. 'I claimed them from Dorothea's shelves—she was always a bad returner.' She watched him turning the leaves of *The Spoils of Poynton*—one of Alan's favourite novels. Inside the cover something was written, and he began to read it aloud, frowning over the cramped italic hand:

'Who is so safe as we? Where none can do
Treason to us, except one of us two.'

Then he saw her name and Alan's and a date—it was the date of their engagement—and closed the book.

'It's a quotation,' she said, turning away. 'Young people were all like that in my heyday,' she added brightly, then felt at once both treacherous and petty. 'When lavender was twopence a bunch, you know,' she added.

Dermot said nothing. He put an elbow on the sill and looked out of the window.

'We *were* like it,' she thought, closing a drawer, having forgotten what he was searching for. 'Charles and Dorothea, Alan and I, our other young friends, in the serious Thirties. We believed that we were safe, that our love, so long as it lasted—and we were certain it would last till death—was its own and our safeguard. We were the lucky ones.'

Then she remembered what she had been looking for and began

opening all the drawers again—from sudden self-consciousness'
Dermot wrongly decided.

'Dorothea and Charles, Alan and I,' she was thinking, '—the
lucky ones.' For the war had soon begun and other marriages were
seen to be not safe, treason was in the air; hazards from outside,
temptations within had done what seemed a lasting damage.

She turned her head and suddenly said: 'Dermot, darling.' Her
voice wavered, rising a little, as if at the end of a sentence.

He looked up in surprise. She slammed a drawer shut and went
over to him and put her arms tightly round his shoulders. He
knew what she was thinking and held her close to him, feeling that
this was the only reassurance he could give.

An unusual lassitude she had suffered lately, Mrs Meacock put
down to the unusual weather. Besides this, moments of doubt—
connected with the menopause, Aunt Ethel would have told her if
consulted—came over her at odd times when her mind should
have been busy with other things. While putting a lattice of pastry
on a treacle tart that morning, she had suddenly looked at her
work with loathing. 'The trivial things I am taken up with,' she
thought, and lifted her head and gazed for a long time out of the
kitchen window at a line of tea-cloths flapping in the wind. She
wondered if she would ever go round the world again, make the
round trip, as she liked to describe it. Alone as she was, she had
nothing if her sense of adventure died. Other people's houses she
was condemned to for the rest of her life, unless she saved
assiduously for her old age, for somewhere of her own—a little flat
over a shop, perhaps. She saw it clearly and was sickened. 'Mrs'
was a courtesy title, she had explained to Kate when she was
engaged. In other days, grander establishments, a cook was
entitled to this. She had never been married. The possibility had
not occurred to anyone else, and hardly to herself. But no one's
going to 'Lily' me, she long ago decided.

Trying to shrug off her mood, she went on with her work. She
brushed the pastry with milk and put the tart in the oven.

'It's only food,' she thought. And will be eaten. And forgotten.

In the afternoon, spurred on by visions of independence and leisure—both the round trip and a cottage in the country—she had taken her box of old cuttings and a pot of paste and scissors and settled on a bench in a warm corner by the south wall of the house. She went through the collection, but found nothing to amuse her. 'I've been so long doing it,' she thought, 'that my sense of humour has changed.' She decided that travel had made her more sophisticated. She even wondered if the anthology would ever be finished. 'This mood will pass,' she told herself. 'It is just like a headache.'

Leaning against the flint wall—it was quite warm, although so early in the year—she closed her eyes, and listened to the birds, and drowsed; and so, when tea-time came, nothing had been done; she had given in to the despair and scorned herself.

Kate came to the kitchen before dinner. Mrs Meacock was quiet and disconsolate, sighed a great deal, kept her eyebrows raised in a dreamy, clownish expression, and when she dropped a blanched almond on the floor, picked it up and stuck it in the trifle, just as if she were alone. Kate, who was feeling self-conscious, glanced about the kitchen and made awkward conversation.

Dermot's way of reassuring her earlier had ended inevitably in love-making. Hastening from him to her duties about the house confused her, and she was sure that evidence was on her face and in her voice, that Mrs Meacock was aware of it and her quiet mood was in consequence. 'If I had walked in with my clothes disarranged, she could not be more aloof,' she thought.

'You'll never stretch the sirloin for an extra three,' Mrs Meacock told her. 'Not with that sort of carving the master does.' It was criminal the way Dermot hacked at a joint, using a saw-edged breadknife, cutting thick steps of meat all ragged round the bone.

Kate had thought it would please Mrs Meacock to hear of Edwina's visit, knowing how much she disliked her and found a challenge in showing her everything done perfectly. She had watched her on other occasions, putting finishing touches to dishes they ordinarily had plain and so obviously thinking: 'We know how to do things here,' as she piped rosettes and brushed beaten egg over everything. But this evening, Edwina's coming seemed only a nuisance; Ignazia's too. That Louisa wanted to invite the Curate was the last straw.

'We had better do some switching about,' said Kate. 'The sirloin could be cold for Sunday supper.'

She leant against the dresser, feeling shaky.

Mrs Meacock, now stirring a sauce at the stove, was able to keep her back turned. It expressed disapproval, Kate thought.

'Shall I get a turkey?' she asked. 'I saw some in the village.'

'I shan't have much time for plucking and drawing.'

'They were done already, and trussed.'

'Then I wouldn't want to answer for it, I'm afraid.'

'We can think about it tomorrow.' Press her any more at the moment, and notice would be given, Kate thought. There had been other times lately when these talks in the kitchen had embarrassed her. Discussions about menus had petered out, as if Mrs Meacock had wearied of Kate's domestic role and refused to go on with the game, realising it meant nothing.

She turned round at last when a sudden movement of Kate's jangled the cups on the dresser. Before she could look away, Kate smiled and frowned at the same time and put her hands over her ears, for in the drawing-room, Ethel and Louisa had struck up—the first dismal bars of *Le Cygne* broke off in confusion and were begun again. Mrs Meacock shook her head slightly, as if she had earache, and Kate, unable to strike any note of friendliness, made the sound of the front door slamming an excuse and went out into the hall.

'And how is my gay little Mother?' Tom asked, leaping upstairs as though pursued by the noises in the drawing-room.

As she passed the dining-room door Dermot opened it, and beckoned her inside. 'We are safe from the music in here,' he whispered. 'I am having my drink peacefully.'

He shut the door behind her and pressed her close to it as he did so.

'It will all begin again,' she thought in a panic, and felt tired and light-headed with desire. She gave him a quick, dismissing kiss and turned away. While he was fetching her a drink, she sank down on the window-seat and closed her eyes, as if she had come downstairs for the first time after a long illness and had found herself too weak for the effort.

'We should leave our love-making till the dead of night,' she thought. 'And bury it secretly in sleep.'

.   .   .   .   .

'What are you doing in here?' Lou asked. There were Dermot and her mother, sitting at opposite ends of the dining-room, so silent that she had thought the room empty until she opened the door. 'I suppose you couldn't bear the noise we were making, but it's really about the only pleasure Aunt Ethel gets. I came to lay the table.'

'You look a bit under the weather,' Dermot said.

'I think I've got a sty coming.' She opened a drawer and took out some knives and went round the table with them, holding a handkerchief to one eye. 'You're sure it's quite all right about Father Blizzard, Mother? You're absolutely certain that you don't mind?'

'Of course. I'll telephone later.'

'He isn't on the telephone.'

'Then I'll send round a little note. Tom can take it.'

'He'll have to push it under the front door. There's no letter-box.'

'Well, he can push it under the door, then,' Kate said patiently.

'He is almost beyond communicating with,' Dermot said, wondering how often Lou had tried to do so, since she knew the obstacles so well. 'All I can say is that I hope my mother won't be in one of her anti-clerical moods.'

Louisa, having laid out the knives, was now groping one-handedly in the drawer for forks. 'Your mother?' she asked, dabbing at her eye and looking dejectedly at him out of the other.

'Edwina is coming for a day or two,' said Kate—in a voice rich with anticipation, Dermot observed.

'Oh, I see,' Louisa said, in a much duller tone. She wished now that she had not mentioned Father Blizzard. All the trivialities, the mockeries she deplored would be made worse with Edwina there, gossiping about what Dermot called 'the fringe nobility'. Earlier that evening, when she had left—been left by—Father Blizzard, she had wondered what she could do for him, how she could show him that not all the village was ranged against him, and on the Vicar's side. An invitation to dinner seemed a poor idea, after all her dramatic daydreams, and she several times decided against it, but nothing better came to mind, and in the end she suggested it to her mother. Kate, who was in her bedroom, looking through some old books, had acquiesced vaguely. Now it was too late to make a change. Dermot, who was touchy about Edwina, would no doubt guess Lou's motive, and be offended. She would be glad if Tom were to lose the note or for Father Blizzard to be called out to some sick parishioner. The responsibility of having him under this roof was too great, she saw; yet, although she was heavy-hearted at the thought of his coming, she was keyed to the prospect now and wondered how she could bear it if he did not.

In the old days, her mother would have guessed what was going on in her head, and found some solution. She had always been one step ahead of events and ready to prevent agonies and embarrassments. Nothing was ever put into words, but they had all known what she was up to and been grateful as well as relieved. At present, however, Louisa realised, she was quite insensitive to the situation, or else she did not care.

'Is there soup?' Lou asked.

Kate nodded, sipped her drink, gazed out of the window.

Ethel, with her 'cello, on her way upstairs, stopped at the open door.

'Oh, you're all in here. Did Louisa and I keep you out with our cacophony? I do wish you had said. You had only to put your noses round the door and we would have stopped at once. I quite thought you were both upstairs. "Come on, Louisa," I said. "We can have a quick scamper through our piece while they're up-stairs." '

Kate said: 'Don't worry. We were perfectly happy.'

'Perfectly,' Dermot murmured.

'All the same, another time . . . it's a fine thing if you are to be kept out of your own drawing-room. Well, hallo, dear boy. Did you have a good day?' She smiled up the stairs at Tom, who was coming down.

'Carry that thing up to Ethel's room for her, Tom,' Dermot shouted.

'Now, please, I am perfectly well able . . . I've dragged it round for forty years or so . . . Be careful with it, won't you, darling? Lou, my pet, your eye looks sore.'

'I feel I've got a sty coming.'

'She needs some yeast,' Ethel told Kate. 'I know you think I'm a cranky old thing, but try to persuade her.'

Kate looked at Lou with such a strange expression, Ethel thought. If it did not denote indifference, it meant nothing at all.

. . . . .

As Saturday went on, Mrs Meacock found herself less and less able to answer for the turkey, and by the time it was too late to buy anything else, was convinced, she said, that it was off.

'I simply can't make up my mind,' Kate said, and then called out to Tom who was passing the kitchen door. 'Come in and take a sniff at this bird, will you?'

'I already have. I really can't spend my day off with my nose stuck inside an old turkey. It makes me feel sick. And I don't know what it's *supposed* to smell like.'

'But did you think it was all right?'

'As right as rain,' he shouted back, and slammed the front door after him.

'It seemed to me he was taking the easiest way out,' Mrs Meacock said.

'What did Louisa say?'

'She thought, as I do, that it has a musty smell.'

'Well, it can't be so very bad if none of us is sure,' Kate said, and called to Ethel, who, although uncertain, inclined towards optimism. 'I should scour it out with salt,' she said. 'Just to be on the safe side.'

Mrs Meacock had already done so, along with other remedies, which she described. 'I'm never happy when my birds come trussed,' she kept saying. 'In spite of the time factor, I would rather have done it myself.'

'None of us thinks there is *much* wrong with it,' said Kate.

Lou, wearing an eye-shield, came into the kitchen and stood watching them, looking anxious and woebegone. Now that she knew Father Blizzard was definitely coming to dinner, she was in despair. At first she had tried to comfort herself by thinking that whatever went wrong, at least the food might be better than at his lodgings, and now it seemed certain that it would not be. And Edwina had arrived during the afternoon in one of her most tiresome moods, full of what she no doubt thought an infectious gaiety, with trilling laughter and up-to-date badinage. Louisa had observed her with one eye, and felt doomed.

'Well, at least the breast will be all right,' Kate said, decisively. 'Edwina will be safe with that. The family can toy with the tainted bits.'

'There isn't only Edwina to be considered,' said Lou.

'Plenty of breast for Ignazia, too. I hope the Curate won't say that it is good in parts. We shall all be waiting for that, I suppose.'

'What an odd collection of people coming,' she thought. She remembered dinner parties in the old days—six carefully chosen guests, and the children in bed, or away at school. It was years since she had given a party like that.

This evening, the collection was to be even more odd than she had imagined, for at four o'clock Sir Alfred's car came up the drive. She had just gone up to her bedroom to fetch a handkerchief and have a little rest from Edwina and was sitting on the window-seat wishing the afternoon away. She wished much harder when she saw her father-in-law standing below and the chauffeur turning the car and driving away again. 'He's dropping in,' she murmured, watching him through the curtains. 'He's sent the car away and he'll stay and stay and Dermot will go mad.'

Before ringing the bell, he stood for a moment, examining the plantains which were growing prolifically in the gravel. Looking for weeds, he had found them. Then he glanced up at the house—and Kate drew hastily back—searching for structural defects and probably discovering those, too, she thought. He was clever at finding signs of neglect—thrips on rose-trees, woodworm, furred-up pipes, choked gutterings. He could catch things in their early stages and give advice, but nobody was grateful.

At last he rang the bell. He always seemed to resent having to do this, for he could not look upon himself as an ordinary visitor and apparently expected someone to have been on the look-out for him, ready to fling the door open as he approached. This never happened, for he was never anticipated; he came uninvited always, as he was bound to in this house, if he were to come at all.

When she forced herself to go downstairs again, Kate found that Ethel—with her usual way of trying to repay favours—had welcomed him and taken charge. The heavy black coat, smelling of cigar smoke, was on the settle in the hall and Sir Alfred was standing in front of the drawing-room fire, polishing his spectacles and making a speech to Edwina about the Stock Exchange.

'Well, Kate,' he said, turning as she came in. 'I've brought up some balance sheets I want Tom to go through during the week-end. I told him to ask me for them yesterday, but no doubt it went out of his head.'

Dermot, sitting on the piano stool, eyed him listlessly.

'I'm afraid he's gone out,' Kate said.

'And, in case I forget to tell you before I go, that creeper ought to come down—it's pulling the plaster from the front wall.'

'*My* front wall,' Kate thought. 'It's so pretty, though,' she said.

He thought she was being obstinate. She would never plant out flowers in beds and borders where one expected to find them;

instead, she let them run riot over the walls of the house, where they encouraged damp.

'I do think Buckinghamshire flint is so beautifully macabre,' said Edwina. 'A dying art, I dare say. The house must be the more valuable because of it.'

'Only if it remains standing,' Sir Alfred said.

Kate saw Dermot turn aside and yawn.

'An estate agent told me once that he can always add a hundred pounds to the selling price of a house if it has a wistaria growing on it,' Edwina said. ' "Wistaria-clad walls" they say when they advertise it.'

'So lovely,' Ethel murmured.

'I remember telling Alan when you first came here,' Sir Alfred said, turning again to Kate, 'about that jasmine, I mean. I warned him he'd regret it, if he left it there.'

'True, that you used to oppress him, too,' Kate thought. 'He always loved it, and so do I. We all do. In the summer it pushes its way in through the windows so that we can't shut them. Such a lovely scent.' She lifted her chin, clasped her hands behind her back and smiled.

Louisa, hunched up, shielding her sore eye, brooded like some sick, imprisoned eagle.

'What's wrong with the child?' her grandfather asked. For some reason, he would not ask questions of the very young.

'She has a sty coming,' Ethel said, and she put one finger under Louisa's chin, stroking her and thinking that she looked pathetic.

'What, is she run down or something?' Sir Alfred asked Kate.

'Your father-in-law was just telling me, Kate, about some wonderful shares he had a tip for,' Edwina said.

Resenting this expression—as a Nonconformist who abhorred gambling—he frowned. 'I had information from my broker,' he explained in a heavy voice.

'Yes, wasn't it marvellous? It came up,' Edwina said. 'The very next day after he bought them. I would never have had such luck. The only time in all my life that I won the Tote Double, you would never guess what it paid – nineteen shillings! Well, and then presently, Sir Alfred, this clever one, sold out, and the minute after they all went down again.'

'It wasn't quite like that,' he said, smiling at her as if she were a child.

'And how much did you win, sir?' Dermot asked, speaking at last.

.   .   .   .   .

Dermot, listening to the anxiety in Kate's bright voice, began to carve. Mrs Meacock had shut the kitchen door and sat among the empty saucepans, wringing her hands. She had basted and sniffed and changed her mind until she was exhausted. Deeply she blamed Kate for the predicament, and, at the very end, had lost her nerve and suggested opening some tins of braised kidneys and making up something with rice. 'Mother never eats kidneys,' Dermot had said. 'And I should be expected to have told you so.' He had come to the kitchen for ice, and had looked all round him and behind the door, saying: 'Surely I can smell that dog of Ethel's?'

He was carving at a side table, which he had removed as far as possible from the big table, and had his back to them all. Tom, who was not above nudging his elbow and muttering comments, carried the plates from him as they were ready. 'I think the stuffing's a mistake,' he murmured, tipping it from Edwina's plate back on to the meat dish. His nostrils quivered. 'I'll forget it, then,' Dermot said. His face was very red. He hated carving at the best of times, and this was not the best of times.

Louisa, holding a handkerchief to her eye, offered brussels sprouts one-handedly.

'Don't forget to give Father Blizzard the parson's nose, darling,' Edwina told Dermot, breaking off for a moment from an argument with Sir Alfred. She had talked to him so incessantly about Victorian furniture that he had taken offence.

'I didn't have the whole of my life in that reign, you know,' he said. 'I know a bit about what's going on nowadays, too.'

'But you probably have some lovely old pieces,' she said.

Father Blizzard, noticing a look of bewilderment on Ignazia's face—for Ethel had been shouting slowly, to make herself understood, mouthing words carefully at her—began shyly to say a little to her in Spanish. His hesitancy embarrassed him, but her expression of interest and relief made him persevere. 'Showing off,' Sir Alfred thought. 'After all, the only reason these foreign girls come here is to learn English—wasting their time to talk to them in their own language, and not very civil to the rest of us.' 'I certainly have a very fine old mahogany sideboard,' he told Edwina in a loud voice.

'And aren't they magnificent? My friend, Lord Auden, and I cut one up the other day. We made a writing-table and two whatnots and a bedhead from it, and painted them all Adam green and white. We had a man sawing away for hours—great fun.'

'Dreadful fun,' he said.

'Oh, no. We never leave things as they are. I mean a completely Victorian room would choke one or make one hysterical. But isolated monstrosities can be amusing and even made quite pretty with a lick of paint.'

'Are you in the business?'

'No, I only help my friend. He says I have a flair.' She glanced across the room at Dermot whose back was turned to her, and then, for Kate's benefit, looked down at her plate as if she were trying to hide a smile.

'Your friend needs to be careful about woodworm, buying old stuff,' Sir Alfred said severely.

'I doubt if he ever gives it a thought. Dermot, where is that delicious-looking stuffing I saw Mrs Meacock busy about this afternoon?'

'She overlooked it. It was forgotten. Just before dinner she came and apologised,' Dermot said, hoping he had pushed it all back inside the bird and out of sight. Kate now looked more put out than ever. She wanted to run away, or get completely drunk.

'What is Ignazia saying to make you look so worried?' Ethel

asked Father Blizzard. 'One can guess quite a lot of Spanish, of course, but I couldn't follow any of that.'

Father Blizzard looked embarrassed. He put his head on one side and appeared to be trying to find a suitable translation.

'I am saying that what we learn at home about the English is not true,' Ignazia said. 'They are not so quiet. I believe they are very quick and indecent.'

' "British",' Ethel said firmly. 'You should say "British", my dear. Otherwise you give offence to the Scots. You don't mind my correcting you, I hope.'

'I have not yet met any Scotsmen,' said Ignazia, 'so I cannot speak for them. Perhaps they are very decent and polite.'

Dermot and Tom, carrying their plates, came to the table and sat down.

'Now, my dear young lady,' Sir Alfred began, 'we can't have you casting aspersions of this kind—'

'She won't understand "aspersions",' Ethel said quickly. 'What other word is there?' She clicked her fingers, as if summoning a simpler word out of the air.

'Calumnies,' Louisa murmured, but only Father Blizzard heard, and turned his head and smiled.

'In Spain we are strict with morals,' said Ignazia, who was not in the best of moods The company bored her and she thought the meat was bad. 'Spanish men wish to have a good girl for a wife. Not as here.'

'These games about national traits are always such fun,' said Kate. 'Won't you have some cranberry sauce, Father Blizzard?'

'Thank you. An un-Christmas turkey is a great treat,' he said. 'And so delicious.'

'And how long were you in England before you began to make these grave charges?' Sir Alfred asked Ignazia.

'You haven't any cranberry sauce either, Ethel,' said Kate. 'Dermot doesn't like it, I know,' she said, conversationally, to Edwina. 'He even refuses apple sauce with pork, doesn't he?'

'I wouldn't give a thank-you for pork without apple sauce,'

said Ethel. 'I like the little extra tartness. And gooseberries with goose. I haven't had that for some time. And grapes with fish, too. Sole Véronique—one of my favourites. Do you like Sole Véronique, Alfred?'

'I am not a fish-eater,' he said, turning briefly from glaring at Ignazia. 'And in that time, my dear young lady,' he continued, 'how many Englishmen have you formed your judgment from?'

Ignazia glanced at Tom, then, seeming to doubt the wisdom of what she had been saying, looked away.

'She's met Tom, for instance,' Dermot said, enjoying this little conversation more than any other part of the meal. Every few minutes, he got up and went round the table with the wine. Glasses remained filled, however, except his own and Kate's and Tom's.

Tom kept helping himself to cranberry sauce, smothering his turkey with it. 'Of course, Dermot and I got the worst bit,' he thought. 'Or so I hope.'

'You must not base your judgment of Englishmen upon my grandson,' Sir Alfred said.

'Poor Louisa,' Father Blizzard said softly to her. 'What a reward for your good works. Perhaps you picked up a germ at the jumble-sale.' He was eating his turkey as if with great enjoyment, and Louisa tried to do the same, but she felt she knew too much about it.

'There are *some* well-behaved, polite young men in England,' Sir Alfred was saying, and he smiled to give the impression—but not to Tom he hoped—of jocularity. 'There are even some who know how to turn up to work on time.'

Ethel laughed uneasily, and Dermot said to her, 'It is always nice to be able to predict when people are going to turn up.' He wore the bland and careless expression that was bound to worry Kate.

'Too bad that it's with early mornings one has to start the day,' Father Blizzard said. The effect of words this evening, he had noticed, was inclined to be explosive and he paused before his remarks with doubt and after them with apprehension.

'I never mind getting up,' Edwina said.

'And, indeed, why should you,' Dermot asked, 'when you do it so long after everybody else? Mother, dear,' he added.

'Courage seems low at that time—and especially in winter, when it is dark,' Father Blizzard said, thinking of linoleum under his bare feet when he got out of bed, and the grey mornings bicycling down to the cold, cold Eight o'Clock.

'I like to be up and about before breakfast,' Sir Alfred said. 'I have never found much hardship in that. When I was a lad I did a newspaper round before I went to work.'

Tom, who had so often heard of the newspaper round, helped himself to some more cranberry sauce, as if he were too much occupied to listen.

'Mornings *could* be nice,' Louisa said to Father Blizzard. Self-conscious in his presence, she dared not break into the general conversation. 'I always have a picture in my mind of breakfast-time in old-fashioned days, with a lovely bright fire and parlour-maids darting in and out with kedgeree under silver covers.'

'And never to hear the sound of toast being scraped,' he said.

'It might have been nice to have lived in Edwardian days.'

'If you had,' Sir Alfred told her, 'you would probably have been one of the parlour-maids, as your dear grandmother was. That's the other side of the story, the other side of the baize door, you might say.'

Edwina closed her eyes for a moment, as if she feared she might faint from boredom.

'You had better stay in the present day with all of us,' Father Blizzard told Louisa. 'We can't spare you.' Her first brief entry into conversation had gone so wrong. He had seen her take the handkerchief from her sore eye and quickly wipe the other.

'I'm sorry to keep jumping up and down,' said Dermot. 'We are a little short of butlers at present.' As he went round the table, he observed the state of plates. Edwina had left her turkey and

Ignazia seemed in two minds about doing so. Father Blizzard had finished his and even wore a look of simple contentment, for which Dermot was ready to forgive him his maddening geniality. 'No great meat-eater,' Sir Alfred muttered, and put his knife and fork together. Ethel had tried to hide most of hers under some brussels sprouts, not realising that this would only make Kate wonder if there was something wrong with them, too.

'How shamed and bored I am,' Kate thought, '—two wretched things to be, and both at once.' Then she looked at Dermot, coming towards her with the decanter, and was gladdened by his smile. 'None of this really matters,' she decided. 'Let us clap our hands and shout ourselves hoarse and throw our turkey bones into the air, to show how little it means, this empty occasion.'

Father Blizzard was worn out already. He had sinus trouble and his head ached and everybody in the room being at sixes and sevens exhausted him. He spent too much of his time smoothing things over and had begun to wonder if it was worth the trouble—the tea parties and the Church socials, family contentions, his own contentions with the Vicar. He had no gift for it. This evening, he had tried for Louisa's sake, feeling drawn towards her—and she would have been comforted if she had known—by everything she herself deplored. This derisive atmosphere she could not thrive in. The love there was in the house seemed fitful, leaving uneasiness. There was no dependable pattern to it; as—he believed—there was unlikely to be without religion.

'My sister liked the bracelet,' he told Louisa. 'I had a letter this morning so full of praise for it that I wondered if I could ever have sent her anything she really liked before. You must have what my landlady calls a "lovely choice".'

. . . . .

In the kitchen Mrs Meacock slipped on a clean white overall and waited nervously for the summons to collect the plates and dishes. At one point, her anxiety had impelled her to go along the passage to the dining-room and put her ear to the door. She could make out Sir Alfred's voice, but not what he was saying, and then

Edwina—sharp and full of affectation, Mrs Meacock thought—asking about the stuffing. Mrs Meacock had overlooked it. Dermot said. She had forgotten and was full of apologies.

Someone else was talking in a foreign language, and Mrs Meacock returned to the kitchen. 'I should have curried it,' she thought, and pressed her hands against her cheeks in a tragic gesture. 'Never again,' she said aloud, several times. Then she pulled herself together and counted the pudding plates again. The Charlotte Russe had turned out perfectly and there was also a Buckinghamshire dish called stone cream. If she ever went on her travels again, she intended to take the recipe with her, to exchange for others in more exotic regions. Its simplicity might have a certain appeal, she hoped. 'I ought to write a cookery book,' she thought. '—A Cook's Tour of Europe'. For ways of escape from her prison she was continually casting round. But the title had come too readily to her mind; it sounded so familiar that she supposed it had been done before, by someone else. Sometimes, she contemplated writing a novel; for, if human nature is the novelist's raw material, as she had often read that it was, she believed she had seen as much of that as anyone, and had certainly struck a rich vein of it in this household. 'It is time for a fresh start,' she told herself, standing in the middle of the kitchen, at the ready, plates polished and puddings lined up. At last she heard the bell and, smoothing her starched overall, went bravely towards the door.

The Return of the Thorntons

4

IT was late spring before the Thorntons came back to the empty house. Charles Thornton's letter, with the plans he had made for returning, arrived while Kate and Dermot were away. They had gone for a few days to the Cotswolds, driving about without direction, tempted down rutted lanes by the long and beautiful names on signposts—and the longer the name the smaller, it seemed to them, would be the grey village they would find lying between the hills. It was a different world from the Thames Valley, although so near to it—less prosaic, more softly coloured.

Separated from their everyday life, as if in a dream, or on a honeymoon, Kate and Dermot were under the spell of the gentle weather and the blossoming countryside. They slept in bedrooms like corners of auction rooms stacked with old-fashioned furniture which would have moved Edwina and Lord Auden to a delirium of envy, and they made love in hummocky beds, and gave rise to much conjecture in bar parlours where they sat drinking alone, not talking much, though clearly intent upon each other. A strangely matched pair, it was thought. The difference in their ages puzzled the country people, who were convinced—by their too positive happiness—of something illicit between them.

It was a Shakespearean spring—his birthday weather, Kate thought, waking on that day and lying quietly on her side, looking out of the open window at the milky morning, the darting birds, the still transparent leaves. It was the longest time of unclouded happiness she had had with Dermot. Removed from their watchful audience—the chorus waiting to comment on and explain their downfall—their love stood a better chance. Each evening they spoke of sending a postcard home and each following day they forgot to do it.

Kate was always glad to wake earlier than Dermot, to lie looking at the gauzy sky, peacefully warm, and knowing that soon, while half asleep, he would stir, stretch out his hand in search of her and then wake suddenly and pull her close to him as if surprised that sleep had overcome him and interrupted last night's love. There were sometimes old-fashioned beds with loose brass that jingled and he would put his hand over her mouth to stifle her laughter and in the morning they would move hastily apart and with guilty expressions sit up to take their early morning tea.

'While they're away, the mice will play,' Aunt Ethel said to Mrs Meacock. She had been turning out a china cupboard and had found the rose-patterned tea service, which she had given to Kate when she married Alan. 'We'll use this today,' she said. 'I've often wondered why Mrs Heron never does—not even once or twice just to be tactful. At one time I thought she must be keeping it for best, but Lady Johnson came and went and we still had the plain service, so I concluded that my niece dislikes it. Well, it would be a dull world if we all had the same tastes. I'll give it a good washing. Would you believe it—there are still some bits of packing straw in the teapot. I wish I'd hit on something she would really have liked. I'm too old-fashioned—I'm fond of pretty things. It will be very nice having everything on the tray matching for once. I was quite ashamed of that old water jug the other day when Sir Alfred came. I'm a silly old woman, but I feel quite excited—it's so rarely that I do any entertaining, and I dearly love being a hostess. And I'll be quite frank with you, Mrs Meacock, my friend is really very grand and well-connected and I'm not above wanting to impress her. You'll enter into the spirit, I know.'

'I've got an apron upstairs that's just the very thing for when I answer the door,' Mrs Meacock said. 'It really is old-fashioned, biscuit-coloured lawn with drawn-thread work. I was in two minds to give it to that jumble-sale.'

She was icing the cakes—for everything had to be very small and dainty, Ethel said—an Edwardian tea-party. She had been quite excited when, the day before, her friend had telephoned, was deciding on rolled bread and butter and drop scones as they conversed.

'My oldest friend,' she explained to Mrs Meacock. 'We were in Holloway Prison together, years and years ago, so I should like to have everything nice.' She did not say why they had been there, but Mrs Meacock had confidence in her and was sure it had been for a very good reason. 'She has come up from her bird sanctuary to stay in London for a day or two on family business . . . she has so many influential friends and relations . . . it quite impresses poor humble me how all their names roll off her tongue. . . . The Duchess of this, the Archbishop of that. It must be important business indeed to drag her away from her shags and gannets. She worships birds, many an injured gull she's given houseroom to. I'm a little nervous of them myself, but we can't all be the same and it's just as well that we are not. It was the strangest coincidence —I had just written a letter to her—I was sticking the stamp on when the telephone rang.'

The letter had been one of her regular ones to Gertrude with a great deal in it about her niece's marriage, in which they both took so much interest.

'It's odd that we have never heard from them,' she said, her thoughts returning to Kate and Dermot. 'Not even a postcard. I haven't the remotest idea when to expect them back, and there are all Louisa's things to be got ready for school.' At one time, she recalled, Kate would not have dreamed of going away during the holidays, but she kept this to herself. 'I suppose they'll just walk in,' she said and thought, 'But not this afternoon, I hope.' 'We'll have the silver spirit-kettle and that cake-stand of my mother's—all the things *they* never bother with. I'll give them a good polishing when I've washed the china. You can't do everything. The cakes look simply delicious. How quickly you knocked them up. I always think one can get through such a lot of work while one's having a good old chatter.'

It was a great day for chatter.

'I think it often happens at the change of life,' Ethel told her friend Gertrude, some hours later. 'A suddenly increased sexual activity.'

'Delicious,' Gertrude murmured, cramming a roll of bread and butter into her mouth, then licking her buttery fingers. She had some unpleasant manners in spite of her good connections. 'Comes later in a man,' she added. 'And causes plenty of trouble when it does. That's sex for you. If everything about it coincides the way it should it's a miracle, when you consider all there is against it. A tease, a good old booby-trap and no mistake. It won't last long with your niece, you'll find, and he being all that younger, the fat'll be in the fire all right, I've always said.'

'It stands to reason,' said Ethel. They hardly listened to one another, each busy preparing what to say at the next pause. They revelled in talking, in using their raw material—the hundreds and thousands of wonderful words, the flow of ideas and opinions. 'I said it at the beginning and I say it now, take away the physical side and what have you there but disillusion?'

'Marriage isn't all bed, let's face it,' Gertrude was saying as Mrs Meacock came in, with some hot scones—an excuse for walking on again in this scene in which only Ethel had a part.

'I dare say that remark coming from an old spinster made your servant chuckle to herself,' said Gertrude, just before the door was shut.

Ethel felt nervous lest being called a servant would make Mrs Meacock put an end to their pretence, take off her apron and prepare to sulk. She had been very proper and respectful with her 'madams' and a lavish use of the third person singular, but they were acting the play for Gertrude, who was not expected to join in. 'We have to be careful,' she said, nodding at the door and speaking in a low voice. 'There are susceptibilities. She is really rather superior.'

'I thought so,' Gertrude said, but she meant superior *in* service, not superior *to* it.

'We call her "Mrs Meacock".'

'It seems odd to me to call a parlour-maid "Mrs". But it's a topsy-turvy world and it doesn't worry me. I'm too close to nature down there in Cornwall to fuss myself with trivialities. My gardener always calls me "Lovey". We're not conventional.'

She was dropping hot butter down her front as she ate a scone and Ethel tried, and soon succeeded, to put an uncharitable thought out of her head. 'We are none of us perfect,' she reminded herself.

After the interruption from Mrs Meacock, they soon settled down again to discussing the family. Louisa, who was out round the village distributing parish magazines, was the next for dissection. 'There's none of her old bounce,' said Ethel. 'She seems bored and antagonistic. Not with me, thank goodness. We've always been chums. But with all the others, I'm afraid. And very run down these holidays—one sty after another on her eye—and very peaky. "You look quite white and spiteful," Tom said to her this morning.'

'They all live under a strain these days, the young people. Over-stimulated. You can't pick up a newspaper without seeing some minx's half-naked bust. The great mammary age, I call it. I was saying to the Duke of Swanford the other evening . . . I always speak my mind with him. . . . "What's wrong with all the men nowadays?" I asked him. "Were they all weaned too soon, I wonder." How he laughed. Then these continental films and strip-teases, and the endless petting. . . .'

'Not Lou,' said Ethel.

'I wouldn't be young for all the tea in China. It's a miracle to me they don't all take leave of their senses. It's obvious they ought to be married, maturing as early as they do these days—eleven or twelve years old, some of these girls, you know. Why, I was fifteen, and I'll depend you were about the same. It wasn't quite the thing to be any earlier.'

'Fifteen,' Ethel repeated, nodding solemnly. 'And I wasn't confirmed till I was seventeen.'

Gertrude picked up her tea-cup in two frail, shaking hands, and drank noisily.

'I doubt if Tom is chaste,' Ethel said in a low voice, leaning forward.

'One thing very naturally leads to another,' Gertrude said, when she had finished drinking. 'As I say, I wonder they don't all go mad. And I blame the sex-mongers myself, not the youngsters. I saw a film yesterday about a brothel and no punches pulled, I assure you. Even I thought it was a bit near the knuckle. It was certainly unsuitable for young people.'

'Did you actually see . . .?'

'The camera men must have. It must have been actually going on, but they work at artful angles, they show a bit here and a bit there and keep fading out. Something has to be left to the imagination.'

There was an unusual little silence; they ate, and stared reflectively at the tea tray. Then Ethel said, 'Louisa, on the contrary, seems rather young for her age. The trouble with her is that she's lost her sense of security. She still misses her father and she needs some supplement to her diet. All those sties breaking out. She's taken up bell-ringing now.'

'It's a wonderful cure for chilblains—or so my nephew, the Bishop, was telling me.'

'Sir Alfred gets them dreadfully,' Ethel said. She looked up as Mrs Meacock again opened the door, and was glad to see that she did not look at all offended.

'Miss Thornton, madam,' Mrs Meacock announced, and stood aside for her to enter.

'Why, Araminta!' said Ethel. 'Such a surprise!' 'But not a very nice one,' she thought. This would put paid to their conversation.

If Mrs Meacock hadn't given the name, she could never have recognised the girl. She had changed beyond all belief. 'This is a young friend of ours—Miss Thornton, Gertrude. And, Araminta, a very old friend of mine—Miss Devaux.'

The girl stepped forward and held out a thin, cold hand to each in turn, then stood gazing down at the tea table—looking like a refugee, Ethel told Mrs Meacock later. Her hair—which had been remembered as light brown, was now a darker, reddish shade and was bound smoothly round her head, and folded at the back in a complicated knot from which a great deal of it had freed itself. She was very pale, and her shaded eyelids seemed too tired to lift up for long the weight of her lashes. She wore a tightly-belted white trench coat, with a great many tabs and flaps and leather buttons.

'It is a surprise,' Ethel said again. 'We had quite given up expecting you.'

'Father said he had written.'

'Then I suppose his letter is on the hall table waiting for Kate who has gone away for a day or two with Dermot.' There was one she had not been able to place, addressed in a mannish hand, with a London post-mark. She wondered why she had not thought of Charles at once. 'Now, do sit down, and join us, my dear, and tell us all your news. Have one of these scones, there's a good girl. You look most dreadfully thin. They must have starved you in France.'

'I eat like a horse,' Araminta said, and she opened her mouth wide and took a large bite from the scone without touching her lipstick.

'You're like me,' said Gertrude.

But a good appetite was all they could possibly have in common, Ethel thought, looking at them in amusement, and wondering if two people could ever have been more unlike. Araminta had taken off her raincoat and had settled down to her tea. She wore a plain, straight dress, the colour of her hair. When she leaned forward to help herself to something to eat, twisted ropes of bronze beads swung out and the top part of her small breasts showed in a loose bodice.

'It won't be long before Tom gets back from the factory,' Ethel said.

Gertrude, with a little cough to engage her attention, winked.

'It does seem funny to be back,' Araminta said, when she had taken the edge off her appetite. Then she could spare time to look about her and refresh her memory. She got up and wandered round the room carrying her cup and saucer.

'As far as I can remember it, not a thing has changed. Oh, there's the dear old Castle,' she said excitedly, stopping suddenly at the south-facing window. 'When you've been brought up on *that*, the ones abroad fail to impress.' Out of a romantic, cloudy sky, slanting light from the setting sun picked out the Round Tower and ramparts. This afternoon, the Castle ridge formed the horizon —a horizon dark blue with trees. On clearer days in summer, the Surrey hills rose up beyond. 'I remember a picnic years ago, with Mummy and Kate and Tom and Lou—she was such a grizzly little nuisance all day and when we got home we found she was covered with measles, so no wonder. We drove in one of those old horse carriages—are they landaus, or what?—You hire them outside the Castle. Through the Park to the Copper Horse we went. It was lovely weather, and Tom kept imitating the driver, who was Irish, I think, and stank of whisky. Afterwards we went to see Queen Mary's Doll's House and then we climbed up the Tower and waved home. We could make out that row of poplars behind the Church—all that way away. I wonder why I remember that day so clearly . . . I'd love to know if Tom and Lou do, too.' She put down her cup and saucer and began to fiddle with the telescope.

'What are your plans now that you're back?' asked Ethel.

'First I'll get Daddy settled in and then I want to do modelling.'

Gertrude raised her eyebrows at such frankness. She had lately seen a most sensational film which had—the advertisements declared—taken the lid off the secrets of this profession.

'An *artist's* model?' Ethel enquired.

Araminta laughed. She was trying to focus the telescope. When at last the trees swam clear before her, she replied, 'No, photographic.'

Gertrude nodded. While the girl was busy with the view they could observe her in detail. Her stockings were so fine that if one had not been badly laddered, Ethel could not have known that she was wearing any. Gertrude, having stared for a long time, turned to her friend and began to mouth something, but Ethel thought this too dangerous and quickly looked away, and this was a good thing, for Araminta suddenly swung round with the telescope to her eye and said 'Bo!'

Into Ethel's mind came the phrase 'Two dear old ladies'. She wondered why, until she realised it was in Araminta's voice she heard it. 'Two dear old ladies,' she might say later to one of her young friends, describing the old-fashioned tea-party she had stumbled on.

She had finished with the telescope and come back to the table and carefully put an iced cake into her mouth. 'I must be off,' she said. 'I'm going back to London tonight. I just came down to see what was to be done—nothing, as far as I could make out. It all looked very neat and clean, I'm sure. Too neat and clean. I dread it rather.'

She began to put on her coat. She was just tying the belt—so tightly that Ethel and Gertrude, watching her, found themselves holding their breath—when Tom came in. This Ethel, although also wishing Araminta to go, had half hoped for. Her conversation with Gertrude would have to be continued by post.

Araminta stood very straight, finished tying her belt and put her hands in her pockets. 'Hallo, Tom,' she said, for he seemed not to recognise her.

'Is that Minty, wearing a wig?' he asked. She smiled. 'You look like a storm trooper in that coat.'

'Such casual manners they all have,' Ethel thought. Gertrude seemed to have begun another tea.

'You haven't changed at all,' Araminta said disdainfully.

'You have. Is that your car outside?'

'Yes, is it in your way?'

'Not at all.'

'I'm just going.' She turned to Ethel and Gertrude in a contrasting mood of warmth and affection. 'Thank you for my lovely tea. I'll be seeing you again and again, I expect. Please give my love to

Kate and thank her about the house. It's been simply lovely.' Her hand was still ice-cold in theirs. At the door, she turned and blew them a kiss with the lightest, most delicate gesture. Then, looking aloof again, she went ahead of Tom towards the front door.

'Can't you stay longer?' he asked. 'Couldn't we go somewhere for a drink? It's only two minutes b.o.t.'

'What does that mean?' she asked, opening her car door. 'You must remember that I have been out of the country.'

' "Before opening time." Won't you?'

'One of these days,' she said, getting into the car.

'Aren't you frozen in that?' he asked. It was a small, open car and her bare hands on the steering-wheel looked blue. She had draped a bright woollen scarf over her head and shoulders and turned up her coat collar. 'As warm as toast,' she said. She gave him a glimpse of a smile before she started the engine and a brief wave as she drove away.

When he got back to the drawing-room, Mrs Meacock was carrying out the tea tray. 'Thank you, sir,' she said, as he held the door open for her. He stared after her.

'*That* was a surprise, wasn't it?' Ethel asked him.

'Yes, what's come over her?' he asked.

'I meant Araminta,' Ethel said quickly. 'I hardly recognised her at first. Such a weird get-up.'

'I didn't see anything weird about it.'

'Sexy, I thought,' said Gertrude, determined to keep up.

'I rather think you're right,' said Tom.

'I'm old-fashioned,' Ethel said. 'I like a girl to look pretty.' She handed round a packet of filter-tipped cigarettes. They lit up, as she and Gertrude called it, and leaned back comfortably, puffing long streams of smoke ceilingwards, with jaws thrust forward.

'Such a leggy little thing she was when I last set eyes on her,' Ethel said.

'And leggy *still*,' said Gertrude, laughing at Tom.

'Any minute now, she'll wink at me,' he thought and when, almost at once, she did so, he looked quickly away.

'Well, I must check up on one or two things,' he said vaguely, and left them.

In the hall he met Lou, radiant—though still sore-eyed—from exercise and good works. In homes all over the village, people were either picking the Vicar's letter to pieces or had thrown it into the wastepaper-basket. She had delivered the message, she felt, and been rewarded when, as she passed Father Blizzard's lodgings for the second time, he was discovered pumping up a bicycle tyre. 'What will happen to this poor parish when you've gone back to school?' he had asked.

'I wish she'd try to look a little more sophisticated,' Tom thought. 'She'll get nowhere like that.'

Sometimes he truly worried about her.

5

AT three o'clock in the afternoon, the damson-coloured sky looked solid above the frail trees. Kate, hurrying out into Dorothea's garden—as she still thought of it—to fetch some dusters from the clothes-line, felt the air so heavy that she almost ducked her head; the sky seemed to come down to her eyebrows. 'It looks like the end of the world,' she thought—the menacing light over the lawn, the dusters hanging so still from the line. She was so much at one with the heavy atmosphere that she could almost fancy her own malaise having come first—creating the oppressive climate. She had been nervous all day, for reasons and in ways she had not been able to analyse. Her stomach twittered like a bird and there was a metallic taste on her tongue.

Just before the sky darkened, a little gale had sprung up and, seeing petals flying past the window, she had gone out quickly to pick some flowers for the drawing-room. Snatching up tulips, with her hair blown over her face, she had felt a sense of doom, as if, tugging unlovingly at the bulbs, she would cause the earth to open up and would be snatched down into the mouldy under-world, a dishevelled, middle-aged Persephone.

Indoors, windows rattled and doors slammed. The drawing-room looked like a stage-set in an empty theatre, threatening some dull suburban play which would never come to life, not even when, at last, the curtain rose and a cockney charwoman muttering comic deprecations came in to answer the telephone. After a time, the wind had dropped suddenly and, minute by minute, the darkening sky congealed.

She hurried indoors with the dusters. Charles and his daughter would arrive in the late afternoon and she intended to be out of the house by then. How he felt about returning to the house she could only guess, but he would want to do so alone with Araminta, she was sure. Apart from that, she was nervous of meeting him again and had decided to do so with her family round her—that evening, when they were to come for dinner and for their introduction to Dermot. Dermot was nervous, too, she knew.

The armchairs looked as if they were sitting up and begging. She took up the cushions and hurled them back into their places, for a less arranged and stagey effect. Then she lit the fire. Waiting for it to draw, she went to the window, and watched some white birds flying slowly past, above the changed landscape. The sky— just before the rain was tipped out of it—seemed to be as charged with anxiety as she was herself. At any moment she knew it must release its load; but her own immediate future was less certain.

A few drops hit the window, then the rain, slanting down faster, whitened, became hard. She could not walk home until it was over and to pass the time she went restlessly round the house, looked into all the rooms again, fidgeting with the furniture, straightening pictures and the towels on the rails. In Araminta's room, she took up—as she had already several times that day—a photograph of Charles and Dorothea, dressed to go to some wedding, caught as they were leaving by Araminta who had probably been impressed by their clothes and wished to record them for the benefit of her friends at school Charles, to oblige his daughter, smiled kindly at the camera; Dorothea looked uneasy in sables she had borrowed— Kate remembered—from her aunt They seemed to be having a fight round her shoulders, jaws snapped on tails in a vicious circle, glass eyes glinting. Dorothea was making a long neck, chin lifted as if to evade the confusion. 'Oh, I miss you,' Kate said aloud, and put the photograph aside and went downstairs.

In the drawing-room, the hail was rattling down the chimney and hissing among the logs, and the fire, losing strength, began to smoke. She looked for a newspaper to hold out across the fireplace, but could find none, only a torn piece of wrapping paper which was at once sucked inwards and burnt, dropping in charred, tinny-sounding pieces on the hearth.

The smoke rolled out into the room, curling up under the chimney-piece, dirtying everything Kate had been to such pains over—the fresh covers and the white tulips and the polished windows. She was so indignant at this act of God that she swore aloud and almost stamped her foot, like a child. The french windows had stuck and she pushed furiously against them, venting her temper. When at last the doors burst open and she nearly fell headlong into the wet garden, she heard above the beating sound of the rain a car's doors being slammed, raised voices and footsteps hurrying across the gravel to the front door. In despair, she turned back to the room. Having opened the door, she had, instead of clearing the air, simply made a track for the smoke across the room, drawing it down from the chimney and out into the garden.

'Oh, I didn't mean it to be like this,' were her first words to Charles, when he opened the door. He came through the smoke towards her and she put her cheek to his, in what she had always thought of as best-friend's-husband kiss. His shoulder, where she laid her hand briefly, was wet, the rough tweed smelt doggy. He seemed to be laughing at her, and really laughed when she said, 'The fire's smoking. It's too bad.'

Araminta came to the door, unwinding her head-scarf. 'Whatever's happening?' she asked. 'Is that Kate? I can't see. Is the house on fire?'

'Come into the hall and let's have a look at you,' Charles said to Kate.

It was dark in the hall and they switched on the lights and Kate looked dazedly at the suitcases by the door, while she made a long explanation about plenty of fires having been lit before without trouble, chimneys swept, and everything made spick-and-span, as it had remained until the very last minute when they had arrived at least an hour before she had expected them.

Araminta kissed her and then took a tissue from her handbag

and began to tidy Kate's face, which was sooty. 'We'll have a cup of tea, if there's any tea,' she said.

'I wanted it to be so nice,' Kate said to Charles as Araminta hurried to the kitchen.

'It's not a tragedy, the fire smoking,' he said. 'And as it rather took my mind off coming into the house again, I am not ungrateful.'

'It seems so odd to hear your voice after all this time.' 'He never could pronounce his r's properly,' she thought.

'I am very glad you are still only twenty-five,' he said.

'*You* haven't changed at all.' His hair was much greyer, though, and they both knew it. He was a tall, heavy man, with a kind, clownish face; his dark eyes looked tired and his mouth had forbidding lines about it until he smiled. 'And I simply can't take in Minty, or believe that's who she is.' She nodded towards the kitchen. 'A completely different person.'

'To me, too. I find it exciting. There is a lot for me to get used to —Tom and Lou, too—completely altered, I suppose. And how is dear Ethel? And Dermot?' he added, coming rather late to him, he realised, and putting an extra note of enthusiasm into his voice to make up for it. Kate, not missing it, thought how very well she knew him.

'It seems strange that we have never met,' he went on. 'That there could be someone so important in your life whom I know nothing about.'

'Yes, I suppose it is very strange.'

Dermot had so rarely come to the house in the days before Alan died—although he brightened, lightened the occasions when he did come, Kate had thought. Her husband had not agreed.

'Dorothea met him, though,' said Charles.

'Yes.' Afterwards they had discussed him in a rather silly, girlish way, and Kate had felt great pleasure when her friend had teased her for Dermot's attentions the night before—some compliments he had paid, perhaps. It was not so odd that she had forgotten, for so many other compliments had come after, in the Irish brogue he seemed to feel appropriate.

'Very good-looking, Dorothea said.'

Kate smiled. 'She looks smug,' Charles decided. Then she glanced up and smiled at him instead of to herself—for the first time since he had entered the house. 'So we can use that name,' she said in a happy voice. 'It is lovely for me to be able to say "Dorothea" again to someone. "If I can't talk about her," I thought the other day, "I'll lose her completely." She was beginning to fade away.'

'We can refresh one another's memories,' he said. 'But has everyone round here—the friends I thought we had—have they all forgotten her, or put her out of their minds?'

'They have put *me* out of their minds, I dare say. I see little of any of them nowadays.'

She did not say why and he did not ask her, and without answering her, he took two of the suitcases and carried them upstairs, and Kate went to the kitchen to help Araminta.

She was standing by the stove, holding out her thin hands over the kettle to warm them. Her nails were long and painted gold. She turned and smiled as Kate came in.

Kate was uncertain of her. The relationship had broken. Since they last met she had gone through the most astonishing and unpredictable change that any human being can make—from a schoolgirl into a young woman. There was something of Dorothea in her—her lightness of step and voice and her neat movements, even a habit of lowering her eyelids and pressing them with thumb and forefinger, as if deeply reflective. She did so now, and yawned—so perhaps, thought Kate, she was simply tired. She was even rather untidy as her mother had been; but her untidiness had style and seemed to be intended. Everything about her was more defined. She was in fact beautiful, and Dorothea had never been that—had only had a gentle charm; and charm—or what that word had once meant—was now an old-fashioned quality, Kate knew.

120

'You've found everything, then,' she said.

'It was all ready. I only had to look for another cup and saucer.'

'I meant to go before you arrived. I thought you would both like to be alone for a while.'

'The very last thing—for *my* part,' Araminta replied. She stood there, guarding the kettle, and a silence fell.

Kate wondered what to say to her, how to begin to discover what sort of a young woman she had grown into. 'Are you in love with anyone?' was what she really wanted answered, but saw that it was likely to be a long time before she would find out. 'Were you happy in France?' she asked instead.

'So happy,' said Araminta. From her tone of voice, and the quick smile that went with it, Kate guessed that even if she had not enjoyed it, she would have pretended that she had; but it was all guess-work now—the child she had seen grow up, her god-daughter (she had held her in church, given presents), the girl handing round tea after the funeral, had been spirited away, might never have been. Instead there was a strange and beautiful creature, turning her hands above the gas-flame, as if weaving a spell; she smiled to herself, watching the gold sparkling on her finger-nails.

It was raining more steadily, falling softly against the windows, and Charles came in to tell them that the fire had stopped smoking and the room was beginning to clear. Water, however, was gush-ing from a choked guttering into the kitchen yard. The house seemed sulky after long neglect. 'I'll see to it tomorrow,' he said cheerfully, and Kate saw him take what he believed was a secret check of the kitchen, a quick glance round to re-acquaint himself. 'He would really have liked to be alone,' she thought. 'Thank you for doing so much, Kate,' he said.

'But Mrs Clarke came in and cleaned it all. "Nine o'clock tomorrow morning," she asked me to tell you.' The kind-hearted woman had hoped to be there this afternoon to welcome them and was not easily persuaded to stay away. 'If only Madam could be here waiting for them,' she had said several times to Kate. She had once worked for Dorothea, and missed her company and the life of the house which she had shared. 'What a home-coming!' She put herself in their places and was made wretched by the situation.

Araminta poured out the tea and they sat down at the kitchen table and drank it. Charles, through the steam from his lifted cup, looked at Kate. It was difficult to decide in what way she had changed. To his fairly unobservant eyes she appeared very much the same. She had put on an old sweater of Dermot's—for she loved to wear his clothes, feeling herself in his embrace whenever she did so. It was loose on her and she had pushed up the sleeves, showing her brown arms. The skin on the elbows was loose and crinkled, he noticed, but most likely had been so for years; she had a few grey hairs. But even if she looked a little older, in some strange way she seemed younger, with an air of uncertainty he associated with, but nowadays never found, in very young women.

She looked up and met his attentive gaze and at once lowered her eyes. She kept her head bent, and turned her cup in its saucer, and ran a finger-tip along a crack in the table-top. 'Do you remember the *fondue* party we had in here—the four of us?' he asked her. She smiled and nodded.

'The cheese went stringy. Poor Dorothea. Alan seeing how far he could stretch it on his fork . . . then lying awake half the night with the pain in his chest and cursing us.'

'Happy times,' said Araminta lightly, as if to two children. She took a small looking-glass from her handbag and briefly examined her face, as if to make sure that it was all there. Then she began to comb her hair. Her father looked at her in a puzzled way. She was a mysterious being to him. Everything she did seemed to call for comment, but so far he had made none. He could no more criticise her than a being from another planet.

In the evening, Araminta wore, precariously, a straight piece of black silk, gathered under her arms and slit a little at the hem to allow her to put one foot in front of the other. Her hair was looped smoothly and demurely against her cheeks in the manner of the young Queen Victoria—Charles, following her into the drawing-room, had his eyebrows raised, as if questioning whether or not, in this attire, she would be allowed to remain. 'Whatever non-plussed means, Mother is looking it,' Tom thought. Dermot had become very Irish, he also noted.

It was Louisa's last night of the holidays and she felt unreal, between two worlds, neither meaning anything. The fact of having guests in the house increased the feeling—something was being set in train which she could not follow. It was hardly worth-while to interest herself in the beginnings of a situation she would soon be snatched away from. She stood back, with one hand on the piano, waiting to be noticed, and when Araminta, passing on immediately after a brief word with Tom, came across the room to talk to her, Louisa knew quite well why she had done so. Older girls invariably did. Thus, they made Tom feel impatient—a good thing—and while he crossly watched them, they could display a generous friendliness and great vivacity to his young sister—the very one they had most wanted to see, their ally, their foothold in the house. Louisa, as usual, glumly responded.

'Minty! What an original dress!' said Aunt Ethel.

And Araminta seemed delighted with Ethel, too, and gaily smiled. Like Louisa, she regarded herself as good with old people. 'I made it my very self,' she said.

'It is most unusual.' But Ethel wondered where any making had come in—it seemed just strung on to a piece of elastic.

'It's hell when I want to pass water, though. I'm bolted in the W.C. for hours and hours. It's so tight round the hem, d'you see, that I have to take it right off.'

'One naturally wouldn't think of that beforehand,' Ethel said bravely.

'It certainly is quite a performance. One always hopes to escape it.' She looked measuringly at the glass of sherry Dermot handed to her.

'So yet again,' said Charles, 'I have to apologise for being late in this house. Once upon a time, it was Dorothea who was un-punctual, and now it is Minty.'

'Oh well, I'm very sorry,' Araminta said. 'At the last moment, I remembered I must shave under my arms.' Turning to say this apologetically to Kate, she split some sherry down her dress. At once, Tom was ready with his handkerchief, and as he dabbed at her skirt, his knuckles brushed against the softness of her stomach, warm under the thin silk. 'My God, she's got nothing on under-neath,' he thought, and felt faint.

Dermot had come without a word to fill her glass from the decanter. 'But there was no need,' Araminta protested. 'I had too much to begin with. I've just been telling them about my difficulties.'

He said nothing to her and at once turned and smiled as Charles praised his dry martini. They were walking in circles round each other, Kate thought—both Dermot and Charles. When she had introduced them, Dermot had shaken hands with an air of boyish respect, almost adding 'sir' to his greeting, and Charles seemed to try to avoid looking at him or showing more than ordinary interest. Although he had not met him before, even as far away as in Bahrain he had heard stories, and Kate, writing to tell him of her marriage, had done so in a defensive strain, as if an explanation were due and she could think of no very good one.

'Do you remember that day we went to Windsor Castle?' Araminta asked Lou.

'I do,' Tom said. 'We went in a carriage through the Park, and you kept waving your hand—pretending to be the Queen, with cheering crowds all along the route.' And very silly she was to do so, he had thought at the time, looking away from her in sulky embarrassment. He could vividly see the picture of himself turning his back, and marvelled at how stuffy he must have been as a boy.

'I can quite believe I did. I used to stand on that little balcony outside Mother's bedroom and pretend it was Buckingham Palace and a great throng down below calling for me. People say they're sorry for Royalty, but I'd give anything to be one of them.

It must be intoxicating. I made up my mind to have a wreath of gold leaves instead of a tiara—beaten very thin and on tiny stems so that the leaves would tremble when I moved my head. I saw the very thing once in a history book.' This was hardly Tom's subject, but he appeared intent upon it. 'I would certainly dispense with all those ghastly decorations and sashes,' Araminta went on briskly. 'That dowdy old Order of the Garter. It makes a clutter of any dress. Sometimes,' she said, with a note of triumph at the very idea, 'I would go to a ball without any jewellery at all.'

'Except for the wreath of leaves,' Tom said.

'Not even that.'

Lou could only keep thinking of the next day—this time tomorrow, she kept saying to herself. The trunks would be piled up on the school landings. She saw it all under a cold light, had experienced it often enough before, the smell of furniture polish, the lists of names pinned to the notice-board, the effusiveness of everyone that first evening. One felt insecure, noting changes— someone's long hair shorn off in the holidays, or Matron wearing a new uniform. This term there would be tennis instead of lacrosse, and her own racquet was ready in her bedroom, with her overnight case and panama hat. After all these years—they seemed a great many to her—she still felt quite shocked and chilly when she saw everything laid out so finally ready. 'I can't remember ever going to Windsor Castle,' she murmured, with half her mind on what she said.

Mrs Meacock opened the door and, catching Kate's eye, nodded and said, 'All serene,' and Charles, so intuitive a guest, at once finished his drink and put his glass upon the tray. Dermot, more lingeringly, did the same, then opened wide the door.

'I shall have a completely *black* habit for reviewing the troops,' Araminta was saying. With tiny steps, she tiupped in to dinner, and 'Lovely din-dins,' she said, sitting down next to Dermot and unfolding her napkin with an air of great anticipation. 'I am always ravishingly hungry,' she explained.

'We are very quiet at our end,' Charles remarked to Kate.

Tom was leaning Dermotwards to share the joke he had with Araminta, who smiled tenderly as she spooned up her soup. The smile was for the joke, but its tenderness for the Vichyssoise, which Mrs Meacock had practised to perfection with her American family.

'Of course; they've forgotten it's my last night's meal,' Lou thought. She had always been allowed to do the choosing before, and it was a tradition that they should have potted shrimps, and cottage pie and tomato sauce out of a bottle, and never any guests.

'You're a comfort to me,' Charles told her. 'When I went abroad, Minty was just like you—a nice English schoolgirl, and I expected her to be exactly the same when I got back. Instead, there is that terrifying creature you now behold. It is too much for me and I shall look at you instead—before you suddenly turn into something else yourself. It must happen under one's very gaze.'

'He tried to be kind,' Lou thought. 'It was not his fault about the cottage pie.'

Tom was pleased that his little story had made Araminta laugh much more than Dermot's had, but he wondered if it were not that she had finished her soup and had more attention to spare, even turning to smile at him, lifting the great weight of her gold-painted lashes to allow him a glimpse of her green eyes. Her head, with its coiled and looped-up hair, looked far too heavy for her frail neck. 'I could encircle it with the fingers of one hand,' he thought, and could hardly endure not to do so.

Tactlessly, Lou thought, Kate and Charles were making plans for later—a visit to some neighbours, others to be asked for drinks —on days when Louisa herself would be gone; half-gone she already seemed. As she listened, she imagined those meetings she would never witness. They looked dull for everyone, sad though she was to miss them.

At every enquiry Kate, Lou noticed, made much of the smallest encounter with her neighbours, trying to hide the fact that she had kept in touch with their old friends hardly any more than Charles had, far away in Bahrain. Her last meeting with one of them—

Lady Asperley—she post-dated at least eight months to Louisa's knowledge and invested with more cordiality than there had been. Lady Asperley, at whose home years ago Kate and Alan had first met Dermot, had been lukewarm about a marriage—disastrous as she believed it must be—for which she held herself responsible. She had known Dermot was a drifter, but his voice reminded her of his father's—a man she had once loved. She liked to close her eyes and listen to it, disdaining the flattery but collecting the beauty of each separate word in her memory. She was a fastidious woman. Charles and Kate thought her like Mrs Gereth in *The Spoils of Poynton*—a novel they had read aloud on quiet evenings in the past—and often called her by that name. From kindness, Kate—so she now explained—did not often invite her to the house. 'Those curtains embarrass her—they are *cotton* damask and she is as shamed by the varnished cabinet in the drawing-room as I am. It actually makes her blush.'

'Who blushes?' Dermot asked.

'Mrs Gereth,' said Charles.

'May Asperley,' Kate added quickly. *The Spoils of Poynton* meant nothing to Dermot, and since Alan died she had half forgotten the name they had once given to their friend.

'We have always thought her so much like Mrs Gereth,' Charles explained.

'I've never met Mrs Gereth,' Dermot said. 'But poor old May, how tedious she is with all her things—"pieces" doesn't she call them? I broke some old china bowl once and I thought she was going to faint.'

Now Kate was blushing, Charles noticed. 'I could never have married a man who didn't simply dote on Jane Austen or Henry James,' she had said years ago. Alan had been the most satisfactory devotee and often talked of Donwell and Pemberley and Poynton—their aspect, the soil on which they stood, the position they commanded—as if he had just recently been staying at them.

'She abhors cocktail parties,' Charles said. 'But sometimes one finds oneself forced to have them, especially in the country, to work people off. Then all the other people see the cars outside and are cut to the quick. I remember May was on one occasion. She didn't want to come, but thought she should have had the opportunity to refuse. The next time, we gave her the opportunity, and she accepted. I remember that Dorothea had one of those raw cabbages with little sausages and things stuck all over it like a hedgehog—it was quite a new idea at the time.' He was now talking especially to Dermot, who looked down at his wine-glass as if he were thinking, 'To hell with the raw cabbage.' 'I was handing the damn thing round on a charger. When I got to May, she looked at it in such astonishment that I suddenly saw how very vulgar and ridiculous it was—this ugly great cabbage stuck all over with olives and onions and things—and bald patches where people had taken things—out of the very goodness of their heart, I dare say. Then I happened to notice a pale, fat caterpillar coming out of the top of the cabbage between a pronged prawn and a piece of mousetrap cheese. He emerged and sat there, staring up at May. I could well imagine how she would talk of that behind our backs—in that lowered voice of hers, even if she were in her own drawing-room and we were safely in ours.'

'She did me at least one great kindness,' Dermot said, at last, raising his eyes and looking at his wife. ('She did it willy-nilly,' Kate thought.)

'But are you working your way up from the bottom or something?' Araminta asked Tom. She put her questions as if in the hope of a long answer to give her peace while she ate. Occasionally, when she had just taken a fresh mouthful or was sipping wine, she looked at him with flattering attention. Her expression was misleading, he decided, for, when he had come to the end of a long complaint about his working life, during which she had lingeringly spooned up her pudding, she said enthusiastically, 'I remember your grandfather well. He is an absolute old darling, I think—' as if she had not listened to a word Tom had said.

When Kate looked towards her and put down her napkin, Araminta obediently stood up. Tottering across the hall with tiny steps, she made for the drawing-room. 'Going up will tear my frock,' she said. 'I simply pray I won't get taken short.' She was combing her hair by the coffee table when Tom came in, her mouth was full of hairpins and she took his hand and pressed one of his fingers to a knot of hair, while she fastened it. 'Thank you,' she said when she had used the last pin. 'My God, I seem to have got scurf again.' She flicked at the front of her dress and cast a look backwards over her bare shoulders. Greatly daring, he brushed a long hair from her back—the most beautiful, narrow, smooth back he had ever seen, he was sure. Too late, he imagined what Dermot might have done—probably asked, 'Do you want this, now, or may I have it?' in a broguey voice and put the hair carefully in his wallet as if it were a holy relic.

Cross with himself and over-anxious with her, he asked, 'Do you have dandruff?' and held the sugar bowl before her.

'Now what are you saying to the poor girl?' Dermot asked. He came over to her with a glass of brandy, warming it in his hands for her. 'Will you just have a breathe of that,' he said, putting it to her nose. She closed her eyes and inhaled, her breasts half-rising out of her dress, then slowly going out of sight again, and went on inhaling as if—Kate thought—it were a bowl of friar's balsam.

'Will she ever look like this again,' Tom wondered, '—in that frock and with her hair like that and the two of us alone?' He wished that Dermot would be done with staring at her bosom. 'This bloody, damned family gathering,' he thought furiously. 'The mix-up of the age-groups, the cramping fools, the this, the that, the rubbishy tedium of it all, with the bloody everlasting chatter, sitting for hours at the table with pins and needles in my feet, all the sodding knives and forks, Aunt Ethel with her surreptitious pill-taking. "Have you seen anything of old so-and-so lately?" "No, old son, I can't off-hand say as I bloody have." '

He spooned some sugar into his coffee and began to stir it. He went on and on doing so, vigorously swirling it in his cup, almost muttering aloud savage phrases, soldiers' words, factory-canteen words, with which he felt at home—until he quite definitely was conscious of a look falling on his hand and raised his head and traced this look back to his mother's eyes. When he had been a child, she had got messages through to him in the same way. He put his spoon back in the saucer. Stirring his coffee for two minutes at a time was one of his Naafi habits, she had told him, and he supposed that she was right. He had soon sloughed off what she had thought innate and her own example had lost its effect. He decided angrily that she was a snob and he was glad that Araminta had combed her hair over the coffee cups. 'That girl and I are made for one another,' he thought.

'Why don't you play to us?' Charles asked Louisa, nodding at the music propped up on the piano—the 'Moonlight' Sonata, with which she was always in deep trouble after fifteen bars.

'Yes, do!' Tom thought. 'That would be nice. That would be very nice. Let's have a pleasant hush and listen to a fugue. I wish I was in a pub,' he mourned, '—I'm so bored that I could cry.'

He stared at Araminta's pointed toes, the buckles on them, one coming unstitched, hanging loose, her inside ankle bones smudged where she had knocked them—from walking with feet so close together, he supposed. 'I wish we were in a pub, both of us,' he yearned. 'That for a start. Really, I hardly know her.' Louisa, having refused to play, sat staring in front of her, as if stunned by the suggestion. 'She makes me feel as old as Polonius and just as stuffy,' Charles told Kate. He looked at his daughter, but could not keep a straight face.

'I can never understand why Polonius has to look so ancient. Need he be quite so tottery on his pins?' Kate said. 'With those youngish children, why should he?'

'He has to look like Lord Burghley, you see. I've no doubt he was made up to be the spit image at the first performance and the idea has gone on ever since.'

Dermot, coming towards them with cigarettes, veered away towards Aunt Ethel. They had seemed, to him, to talk all the evening of people he did not know. It was understandable, he told himself, that they should like to do so. A time would come when the gap was filled and the questions asked and answered and then he would be able to join in the conversation, too. They did not mean to be exclusive, he was sure.

'Now, do sit down, dear,' Ethel said. 'You're too attentive, as usual.' She was enjoying her first cigarette of the day. She always looked forward to it, she told him—and to her nightcap, she added, in a jolly, but confidential tone. She puffed and sipped alternately. Calling a drink a night-cap made it sound medicinal, Dermot thought. 'Another night-cap?' he asked Tom. Not waiting for an answer, he turned and poured one out for himself.

'Mother, would it be all right for me to go to bed?' Louisa muttered, standing by Kate's chair and putting a toe round the outline of a rose in the pattern of the carpet.

'Of course, darling. Just give Charles a kiss and slip away and I'll come up later.' 'It is her last night at home,' she thought, 'and no one but Charles has made a fuss of her.'

'A kiss!' Louisa thought. '*Used* I to kiss him good night?'

'Good night, Lou dear,' he said. He stood up quickly and opened the door for her and wished her a happy term as she went out.

'We don't kiss then,' she thought, 'but he opens doors for me now, instead.' She was grateful for this.

It was gloomy upstairs. Everything looked unfamiliar, especially her own bedroom. When she switched on the light, she saw first of all the ugly panama hat lying on a chair. She hoped that she would not see Father Blizzard on her way to the station in the morning—although she would carry her hat, she would have to wear her grey flannel summer coat. Her room she intended to leave in its state of disorder for someone else to tidy up. They would all be too sorry for her tomorrow to criticise. Most of the drawers were half open and she had thrown things at the wastepaper-basket, not into it, and some of her precious notices were hanging loose from the wall on one drawing pin. Her photograph of Father Blizzard was safely between the leaves of her Bible at the bottom of her trunk. She had taken it herself in the graveyard at a funeral. This had seemed the only chance she would ever have when he would be both out-of-doors and unobserved, and she had stood well back behind the mourners, hidden behind a gravestone. It was not a good photograph, for it was taken against the sun, and there was not much more of Father Blizzard than a blurred white surplice blown backwards by a fierce wind. 'It will do to be going on with,' she consoled herself.

She had packed her hunting-horn too, and the old ear-trumpet. There would be reckless fun next term, she had decided; and thinking of that, could not feel much reality about this dull room where, in transit, she must pass the night. Far more clearly she saw the dormitory at school with its white paint and faded William Morris wallpaper of willow leaves.

She had said good-bye to Father Blizzard that afternoon, and had needed all her courage to go up the little pathway at his lodgings, past his bicycle propped against the railings, to the tiled porch where she had knocked timidly on the door. He may have seen her from the window, for he came himself to let her in, napkin in hand, opening the door to let out the smell left over from cooking. Seeming pleased to see her, he led her into his sitting-room, where a cloth was spread across one end of the table at which he had been eating a late luncheon—owing to an awkwardly timed funeral—of some dried-up meat and gravy that his landlady had kept warm for him. He seemed to be tucking into the meal with humble gratitude and, as he talked to Louisa, cleared it all up and began on a dish of rhubarb—over-stewed into a stringy acid-pink tangle. The sight of it seemed to roughen Louisa's teeth and she had run her tongue over them, shuddering.

Now, as soon as she had said her prayers and got into bed, she would go over the conversation they had had. It had not amounted to much, or gone on for very long. He was imitating the Vicar—a reproof he had suffered from him that morning—when the landlady came in with two cups of tea. 'Must pull our socks up, y'know. Not on the ball of late, eh?' he was saying, in the Army chaplain voice to which the Vicar reverted for the scolding of Curates. The landlady, rather grudgingly, handed Louisa a cup of tea. She had said nothing to either of them and Father Blizzard had made faces at the door when she had gone.

Louisa, trying to keep her mind on her prayers, finished them hurriedly, hearing her mother coming upstairs.

'You're soon in bed,' said Kate. She was just about to comment on the state of the room, but then remembered it was Louisa's last night. Tears, on these occasions, had never yet been shed, but were in the air; infectious, too, like yawning. She was endangered herself. 'I'm very sorry they had to come this evening,' she said. 'There was nothing I could do about it.'

'It didn't matter to *me*,' Louisa said, closing her eyes for a moment. When she opened them again, she saw that Kate, staring listlessly at the untidy chest of drawers, looked sad. Her forehead was quite lined, Lou realised with surprise. The grey hairs she had noticed from the start. 'I'll clear up everything before I go to-morrow,' she said, suddenly not wanting the disordered room to be added to her mother's cares.

Kate bent down and kissed her. 'There's no need,' she said. 'Ethel won't mind doing it. I can't bear to come in here myself when you've just gone. It makes me too miserable, but perhaps Ethel won't be so foolish.'

Louisa put her arms tightly round Kate's shoulders. 'Thank you for the nice evening,' she said. 'It was better than the old cottage pie. I've grown out of that, I think.'

'We've made too sad a dish of it.'

'Didn't Minty look a fool?'

Kate could not answer. Her throat contracted and she was not sure enough of the voice. When she was, she said, 'I'd better go back to them.'

'Will you turn off the light, please?'

As Kate did so, she said, 'God bless you, darling. Sleep well.'

Lying in the dark, Louisa wondered why she always asked that of God, not believing in Him, and then she added a rider to her

133

own prayers, 'Bless *her*, too, please God, as I said before, and don't let her grow old-looking if she doesn't want to.'

She always framed these requests slowly in her mind, as if dictating to an inexperienced secretary.

'We must go,' Charles said, when Kate came down. From knowing her a long time, he guessed that on her way downstairs she had been forcing back tears.

'No, must you?' she said automatically, sitting beside him on the sofa again.

Ethel was pretending not to be yawning, bending down to fondle her dog or pursing and patting her lips in a thoughtful way, as if Araminta's descriptions of meals she had eaten needed her utmost concentration. Her lids blinked over her watering eyes.

'Poor Kate,' Charles whispered, leaning towards her to light her cigarette. 'What do we get out of it, I wonder—being parents?'

'It was great fun when they were little,' she said. In her mind she suddenly saw the three of them, Tom, Minty and little Lou— running naked in and out of the sprinkler on the lawn. It was the memory of a memory by now—the hallmark of happiness, that scene. The sun had shone through the dazzling aigrettes of water and made rainbows, the breeze caught them and fanned them out, and the children leapt and screamed and stamped footprints on the soft, squelching grass. It was a long summer's afternoon and it stood for all the others now. There had been many. And she and Dorothea were together day after day. Their friendship was as light and warming as the summer's air.

'It's a pity about love,' she said. 'The pain one pays for it with— children, or one's friends. It can't be helped.' She shrugged, impatient with herself, but seeming to him impatient with love.

He stood up to go, looked at his watch and then at his daughter. 'She's had a long day,' he said; he, too, struggling not to yawn.

Araminta, however, looked perfectly fresh. As bright as a button, Ethel thought, admiring the way she came to her feet, so straight, so quickly, her fingers laced round her empty brandy glass, looking like Hebe, so young, so full of vitamins.

'Do you know that I could circle your neck with just one of my hands?' Dermot asked Araminta and, spreading his fingers round her throat, almost did so.

The moment they had gone, he went back to the drawing-room as fast as he could and was already pouring out some brandy when Kate came in. He said, 'I'll have another little drink now that at last they've gone. What a mercy I behaved myself so well.'

'Why do you say that?' Kate asked, looking at the ring of cigarette ash scattered round Araminta's chair.

'You were thinking it.'

'Of course not.'

'A very smart pretty girl, Araminta.'

'I think Tom thinks so.'

'Won't you have a drink?'

She shook her head, too tired, suddenly, for words. She went to the door, then, tired as she was, lingered there, compelled, before she left him, to ask what he had thought of Charles.

'A jolly nice old codger,' he replied.

[6]

Tom was wasting the long summer's evenings. Although bowing himself out of the relationship with Ignazia was a constructive activity, it took up very little of his time and gave him no satisfaction at all. The really constructive plans he had in mind made almost no progress, for Araminta was studying at a school for models in London and when he—as he so often did—found himself near the station as she came from it in the evening—walking so quickly, her head high as she gratefully sniffed the May-scented country air—she was always very tired, she said, and, getting into her little car, she would wind a scarf round her head and wave and drive off homewards. Thinking how far from tired she looked, he would watch her until she had turned out of the station slope into the main road. She wore very short gloves and her hands looked like two little white paws on the steering-wheel.

Only once had he persuaded her to stop for a drink with him on the way home, and she had spent the time following The Rake's Progress along the walls of the bar and out into a passage and half-way up the stairs, her nose close to the glass—he wondered if she were short-sighted. She was quite absorbed by the prints and ignored all that he said to her. With a glass of Guinness in her hand, still wearing the white gloves, she took a sip each time she stopped at a picture and when she came to the last one, drained the glass and held it out to him. Even with a moustache of froth she looked delightful to him. 'Delicious,' she said. 'My favourite thing of all.' But she must go at once, she added. That very second she had to be off. 'Just one more drink,' he pleaded. 'No, I am far too dirty,' she said, and examined the spotless gloves with great distaste. Getting into her car, she thanked him for the Guinness—

136

too enthusiastically, he thought, as if it were the drink and not the company that had pleased her. She raised her hand and almost touched her lips with it, blowing him a kiss. 'So sorry I am such a broken reed,' she said, and then had driven away.

On another evening, he called on her with a message for her father which he had persuaded Kate not to telephone. Araminta was watering the garden, for there had been a long dry spell. The sprinkler was turning on the lawn and she was trying to drag it to another place without shutting off the water. Her feet were bare and the front of her dress was wet, the thin stuff clinging to her thighs like marble drapery. 'She will drive that young man mad,' Charles thought, watching Tom's face as he approached. He led him indoors for a drink, and very soon Araminta, having fixed the sprinkler the way she wanted it, came through the garden door to join them. Her feet were wet and little bits of grass were stuck to them. Tom looked at them carefully as they crossed the carpet. 'Another part of her I've seen,' he thought.

She picked up a half-eaten apple from the window-sill, finished it with big, curving bites, then went to the door and tossed the core high across the garden. She flicked her wrist and bent back her elbow as young boys do, throwing stones into a tree; but immediately after, she turned and came back across the room with a gliding walk as if she were on castors. She raised her arms, threw back an imaginary garment from her shoulder, touched an imaginary necklace on her breast, moving with eager impatience, like a race-horse held back, going down to the starting-point; yet she covered no distance. 'This is a mink coat I am dragging along the ground behind me,' she said, and glanced backwards contemptuously. 'It is lined with gingham just for the hell of it.'

'Do you learn this at the school?' Tom asked. He had often wondered what she did there, but she was always vague and evasive about it. She became so now. 'Oh that, and much, much more,' she said.

'Excuse me for a minute or two,' Charles said, not saying, not knowing where he was off to. 'Give Tom another drink when he's ready for it.'

Araminta sat down on the sofa and kept her eyes dutifully on Tom's glass, as if to be ready to spring up the minute it was empty. Tom, coming close to her to offer her a cigarette, smelt the wet cotton dress and thought that she was beginning to steam faintly. 'You'll catch your death,' he told her, bending over her to light a cigarette and look down her bodice. Not knowing how long Charles would be away, he said in a rush, 'I swear your eyelashes have grown longer every time I see you.'

She lifted them slowly, as if with an effort. 'I want to give you a surprise,' she said. 'You must close your eyes and hold out your hands. Now, wait till I say "open". You aren't to cheat. You always did when we were children. *I* used to see you, peeping round the tree when you were supposed to be counting a hundred and not looking. "He'll come to a bad end one of these days," I used to tell myself.'

'I wish we could play hide-and-seek nowadays.'

'There aren't enough of us. You can open your eyes now.' She sat back on the sofa, looking up expectantly, waiting to laugh at him.

In the palms of his hands she had put her false eyelashes, and he stared at the little strips of fringe with exactly the baffled expression she had hoped for.

'And now look at me without them,' she said.

'There's no difference. But what a horrible thing to do.'

'Oh, I do worse than that.'

'Doesn't it hurt most dreadfully?'

She laughed and she took the lashes from him and put them in an ash-tray. When Charles at last came back, he bent down and examined them with curiosity. 'They are Minty's false eyelashes,' Tom explained. Minty herself had dashed into the garden to move the sprinkler again.

'I shall be sick,' Charles said. 'It reminds me of that brace she wore on her teeth when she was small. She was always leaving that lying about.'

Since that evening, although the ones that followed were so warm and long-drawn out and so exactly suited to romantic excursions, Tom had seen no more than glimpses of Araminta. Letting Ignazia down lightly was a tedious exercise, though a matter of principle to him. In every minute of his spare time, he told her, he was taking a postal course in Accountancy. His grandfather had previously threatened this and more recently hinted that he should insist upon it, and Tom had had to play for time with what he thought of as a non-committal agreement. The idea had filled him with the kind of anxiety he suffered when he woke in the night from dreams of being back at school or with his National Service to do all over again.

'It's a free country,' Dermot was always telling him. 'Surely he can't expect to dictate to you about your leisure? He pins you down all day. Isn't that enough for him?'

These conversations were usually above the noise of bullets striking off rocks and the thundering of horses' hooves, for Tom—at a loose end—had made the first payment on a television set. 'Why can't you read a book instead?' Kate asked him. She disdained such ways of passing time, not realising that she very seldom read herself these days and was just off for an evening in the pub with Dermot. Tom kept the television set in his bedroom and he and Dermot liked to sit there with curtains drawn against the sunshine, watching cowboy films. 'Too good an evening to waste out of doors,' Dermot would say, taking a last glimpse out of the bedroom window while the set was warming up—Ethel's dog lying on the hot gravel down there, a column of gnats dancing in the shaft of light under some trees and high above the trees some cirrus clouds paling and dissolving. 'Right!' Tom would say, drawing up two uncomfortable bedroom chairs. On the screen, rods of light ran blindingly into one another, the picture steadied until they were able to see a packet of soap powder capering on tiny legs, singing a ditty. It then took a dive into a washing-machine, and a head of jostling bubbles, singing too, rose up. Dermot darkened the room, shutting out the scent of jasmine, and he and Tom sat down, entranced.

Sometimes Ethel joined them, looking in with a trivial excuse, begging them not to stir and lingering to watch, but as if her attention was only momentarily caught. After hovering for a while, she gradually merged into the shadowy background and was forgotten, until at last, with sick-bed caution, she tiptoed away. Like hares before a serpent, Tom and Dermot sat rigid and in silence. From time to time, their hands groped on the floor for their glasses of light ale, their cigarettes burnt to their fingers.

'You've got to *sleep* in here, Tom,' Kate said crossly, flapping at the smoke-haze with her handkerchief. She had come to find Dermot, who at once stood up and seemed to be on the move, just temporarily detained like Ethel. He walked backwards to the door watching the villain bursting out of Nolan's Saloon with a revolver in each hand.

'Your mother is on the telephone,' Kate said coldly. 'She said "Hallo, stranger", to me, so I'm warning you.'

Dermot went down to the hall. 'Hallo, stranger,' he said, lifting the receiver. 'Well, *you* haven't either,' he added after a pause. 'What have I said so far that's rude? Well, I'm sorry, Mother, but whatever I do is wrong. . . . To hell with Wilfred Auden . . . I think you let *yourself* down over that . . . It was nothing of the kind. I simply changed my mind.'

Kate passed him and received the frown he intended for his mother. The front door was wide open and she stood there in the sunshine, watching Ethel's dog rolling on the gravel. The scent of jasmine reminded her of other summers and she pulled a sprig of it off the wall and twirled it in her fingers, her mind straying over the past and—for all its imperfections—her contentment in it. Not much of it did she want undone. Her dissatisfactions seemed in the present and with herself. She had time on her hands, as Dermot had, and sometimes found it dispiriting.

'I may have other plans,' she heard him say. He spoke very

pompously and, looking across the hall, she saw that he was standing to attention now. 'I may have other plans,' he said again. Edwina was obviously not listening to him.

Kate went slowly across the lawn and sat down on the seat under the monkey-puzzle tree. It had a pattern of wrought-iron bracken leaves and, although dilapidated, had been much coveted by Edwina. From behind the drawn curtains of Tom's window came galloping-horse music and the singing ricochet of bullets. 'We're all of us just passing time,' she thought, feeling irritated by the sound. A lack of purpose was an imperfection Dermot may have introduced. It seemed to her that it was worse for herself, without religion, to be squandering her life, expecting no other and chilled by the passage of time.

Charles Thornton carrying something in a paper bag came through the gate. He was going briskly towards the house when he saw Kate and altered course. She was sitting sideways with an elbow on the back of the seat and her hand covering her closed eyes. Hearing him, she uncovered them and hurriedly shifted to a less dejected attitude.

'You looked like a mourning woman on a tomb,' he said.

'Well, Dermot is quarrelling with his mother on the telephone and I was waiting for him to finish.' Even from where she was sitting, in a brief lull from upstairs, she could hear what he was saying. He was threatening to ring off, but did not do so. 'An expensive call,' Kate said. 'She must be needing the quarrel very much.'

Holding out the paper bag before he sat down, he said, 'Morello cherries, which I knew you like. Do they often quarrel?' he asked, nodding towards the house.

'They do sometimes,' she said vaguely, taking some cherries from the bag. 'So pretty,' she said, holding them up in the sunlight. 'And so delicious,' she added, when she had eaten some and spat out the stones.

'Too sharp for me. I prefer the Early Rivers. Is she possessive?'

'Edwina? Only interfering, really.' He always *had* wanted to

141

know all he could possibly find out about people and his interest surprised her, for men so seldom have it. 'She *will* try to get jobs for him,' she added, wishing to be helpful to him in his efforts to understand, to see Edwina for what she was and her son for what he was to her.

'Is that . . . ?' 'A bad idea' he had been going to ask. He groped for a better, a completely different, ending to the sentence and found none. To Kate, the words were as good as spoken and she pushed the bag of cherries aside and sat in silence, holding the sprig of jasmine to her nose and staring down at the grass. She was blushing.

'In Athens, children bring little bunches of that stuff—jasmine—round the café tables,' Charles told her. Greece, all that way away, must surely be safe to talk about, without the pitfalls of most of their conversation. Knowing himself to be inquisitive and tactless made the traps seem worse when he had fallen into them. 'So many flowers in that country,' he went on, meaning to fill in the pause with some descriptive travel talk. 'Everywhere you go, people always loaded with them, taking them as presents to other people who already have plenty, or trying to sell them—even from one island to another—enormous men standing up in caïques with their arms full of arum lilies, old men with carnations tucked behind their ears, or pinned to their caps. You'd love it there, so many surprises.'

She seemed to have forgotten him. 'Alan was the one who wanted so much to go there,' she said. 'But he was always too busy. We didn't even get to Rome.'

Charles, too, recalled how busy he had been, but this seemed a dangerous memory to revive.

'*I'm* forgetting what it is to be busy,' he said. 'I'm not sure if I like so much leisure—placed as I am. With so much time to spare, there seems to be no reason for doing anything at all.'

'When your leave's over, will the company send you somewhere else?'

'I don't know.'

'The *company*,' she thought. It had featured so much in Dorothea's plans and forebodings. Would the company send them here or there, uproot them, ruin home-life and friendships? She had imagined a set of malignant board-room men taking names out of a hat. 'Thornton,' one read out. 'Gold Coast,' said another.

'What's that noise?' Charles asked, glancing up at the house.

'Tom's television.'

'What an extraordinary thing.'

'I suppose you mean, "Has he nothing better to do on an evening like this?" Well, I dare say he would very much prefer to spend it with your Minty.'

At this, Charles looked smug. He gazed, smiling dreamily, at Ethel's dog, as if it were the rosy future, and he made lathering movements with his hands, leaning forward, his elbows resting on his knees. Kate, sitting sideways, watched him aloofly; then, hoping to convey to him that she was bored with the sight, began to examine her finger-nails instead. Dermot at last rang off. They heard the faint ping when he replaced the receiver. He did not appear.

'Has he gone off to seethe?' asked Charles.

'He doesn't brood on things,' Kate said. This was untrue, but a deserved rebuke to Charles, she felt.

'I'm glad to hear it,' Charles replied, as if relieved that Dermot had one fault less than he had attributed to him.

'You don't understand him. He is too much unlike you. He comes from a different sort of world.'

'A different age group, certainly—from mine, that is.'

Her mood changed. 'I somehow wish you would try,' she said, turning her face from him.

'My dear good Kate if he makes you happy, he is the most admirable person in the world to me—the one I owe the most to.'

'It is his air of indifference—of not being committed . . . it antagonises people. Though I shouldn't say an *air* of indifference. It's real enough. He suffers from melancholy.'

'And has all the time in the world to do so,' Charles thought.

'In the war, you know, his plane was shot down over the Channel. There were four of them in a rubber dinghy for five days, drifting about, lost, in icy weather. The others all had people they loved at home and the thought of their anxiety for them made matters that much worse. They began to despair. Dermot, having no one so precious . . . his mother, of course, but you've heard how he can quarrel with her, or his elder brother he could never bear . . . he had nothing, no one to sap his courage. It works that way, doesn't it? "He that hath wife and children hath given hostages to fortune." Dermot *hadn't* given them. He had made up his mind that he never would. And besides, without the impediments, he saw that he must be brave, for the other three, who had made all those extra difficulties for themselves. His calm was real, not conjured up and fluctuating like theirs. He managed to keep them going. Perhaps his indifference . . . and the underlying melancholy . . . saved their lives. He was only a boy, too. He had just left school.'

Charles nodded solemnly. He wondered how she knew all this.

Dermot at last came out of the front door. He shaded his eyes against the sunset, not seeing them under the tree. He was humming 'The Wild Colonial Boy'—not a good sign, Kate had long ago realised. 'Paddy M'Ginty's Goat' was his fair-weather singing.

'Ah, there you are, then,' he shouted, with false and Irish bonhomie. 'In solemn confabulation are you, now?' He came across the lawn.

'Kate was telling me about your nasty experience during the war,' said Charles.

Dermot looked quickly at Kate, who was busily eating cherries from the bag. 'Why?' he asked.

'It just cropped up,' she said.

'Pretending to be modest?' Charles wondered, as Dermot frowned. He bent down and carefully pulled a blade of grass and sucked it. 'How is Lou?' he asked when he thought the silence needed to be broken.

'She writes her usual Sunday letters,' Kate said. 'All under-linings and exclamation marks. One gets breathless reading them. So unlike Lou, really. Letters from a stranger they seem to me. And exclamation marks always give an air of straining after vivacity. I wonder why she strains for an effect with me.'

'She's happy there, surely?'

'I do hope so. How can one tell? From Tom's Army letters, one would have thought his National Service the happiest days of his life.'

'And so they may have been,' said Dermot.

'Were you in Bomber Command?' Charles asked, looking up at him.

'Yes, old boy,' said Dermot, simply to annoy him. He observed Charles's reaction and then added, 'for my sins.'

'I have some new Vivaldi records,' Charles said to Kate, as he stood up to go. 'You must come and hear them. Both of you.'

'That would be lovely,' she said vaguely. 'Thank you for the cherries.'

Dermot walked with her to the gate to see Charles off. When they turned back, he said, '*Why* were you raking up all that about the war? It couldn't possibly have cropped up. It was more likely dragged in. And what were you saying, anyway? Why do you always try to justify me to him? It isn't the first time. "You may have a low opinion of him, but he has his good points all the same." I can hear you saying it and see him listening to it. Does it matter so much what he thinks of me? *I* don't care—if you're considering me.'

They entered the hall. As Kate passed the telephone she took off the receiver and handed it to him. 'Talk to your mother again, if you want to quarrel,' she said. Going upstairs, she could feel his look of fury between her shoulder-blades. Her calm, prim manner lasted only until she had closed her bedroom door, and then she heard him starting up the car and she went quickly to the window. At the gate he hooted loudly and drove out on to the road.

She sat down on the window-seat and put her hands over her

face. A tear dropped into her palm and ran down her wrist. 'You look like a mourning woman on a tomb,' Charles had said earlier. 'I wish he had stayed,' she thought. 'I wish he were with me now.'

. . . . .

Dermot sat in the village inn, staring at the ribbed wood of the trestle table in front of him. It was not a fashionable place and was empty now except for two creaky old men and the landlady, who rested her arms and bosom on the bar and gazed out of the open door at the village green as if she were in a trance. From time to time, one of the old men would throw a remark at the other, later it would be returned. The atmosphere was dull and slumbrous and Dermot was left in peace to brood over his grievances.

Lest Kate should ask him what his mother had been saying, he had gone upstairs to avoid her as soon as he rang off. 'A few home truths,' was no doubt how Edwina would have described her part of the conversation. Very distasteful he had found them, especially the ones she had delved out of the past—still harping on the money she had lent him on the day when he had promised to go to see Lord Auden. 'Which, I see now, you had not the slightest intention of doing.' ('Oh, I wouldn't say that,' he had replied.) In spite of everything, she could not resist giving him one more chance. He had scarcely listened to her new proposals; had hinted at having other plans, but was not believed. 'Other plans I most certainly have,' he now told himself firmly.

While speaking to Edwina, he had seen Charles coming up the path and had felt in no hurry to meet him, either; so he had lingered upstairs. Taking a book from Kate's bedside table, he had lain down on the bed to read for half an hour. It was one of the novels she had brought back from the Thorntons, the one Alan had given her on the day they were engaged, and Dermot glanced again at the inscription inside the cover:

> 'Who is so safe as we? Where none can do
> Treason to us, except one of us two?'

The uncertainties he always felt on beginning to read a book were

146

increased. He turned the page. '*The Spoils of Poynton* . . . **Preface**' . . . *that* he skipped . . . 'Chapter One'. His expression fell into lines of great boredom as he began to read. 'Mrs Gereth had said she would go with the rest to church.' He frowned, closed the book with his finger in it to mark the place and stared up at the ceiling, wondering where, lately, that rather unusual name had cropped up. He associated it with Charles and then with his friend, May Asperley. It was Charles who had said those two were alike, and he remembered searching his mind for anyone he knew who was the least like Lady Asperley. 'I've never met her,' he had said, having gone through most of the village in his mind.

Recollecting that scene—they were all at dinner downstairs—it was coming clearer to him—his irritation swerved suddenly into anger. Mrs Gereth, then, was simply a character in a book and no one had liked to tell him so. They had preferred to gloss over his ignorance. Charles, having mistakenly assumed (it was their first meeting) that Dermot shared his wife's enthusiasms as Alan had done, had no doubt changed the conversation to cover Kate's embarrassment. And if she were not embarrassed—and why she should be, Dermot could not see—Charles would have put the idea of embarrassment into her head, as if implying that there was some awkwardness in not having read every novel that ever was written and having the names of the characters at one's finger-tips.

Dermot had thrown the book across the floor and a pressed violet fell out—and dropped to pieces, he was glad to see.

Brooding on this, he sat for a long time in the dreary pub, to punish her.

7

'THE mistake she made,' Ethel wrote, 'was to lose sight of the sort of woman she really is. A typically *English* woman, I should say—young for her age, rather inhibited (heretofore), too satirical, with one half of her mind held back always to observe and pass judgment. This temperate climate has its effect—ripeness comes slowly and all sorts of delicate issues find shelter to grow in and so confuse the picture. In Mediterranean countries as one knows, the sun brings girls to maturity much earlier—and I have my own theory that the Vitamin E in ripe olives has a *stimulating* effect on the sexual organs. So different here . . . The weather enervating. Today, for instance, though quite hot, the clouds are very low. One's spirits in accordance. Kate's in particular. (There was a little *contretemps* last night.) Love, for her, should begin in the *mind* first. I remember her courtship with Alan—a different matter indeed— the evenings at the Queen's Hall (the dear old place!) and the long hikes, as people used to call a country walk, and the books going to and fro with passages underlined. The marriage of two minds it most certainly was. He left a blank that no one (?) can fill, and what a pity that she didn't face the fact. Better for Dermot too if she had. She could have made a good enough life for herself out of what was left, and had started to do so, then Mr Wrong came along. How disastrous for him that he ever did! At an unsettling time for *her*, too. At the age when many a woman feels restless and un- wanted, still feels young inside, grey hairs notwithstanding. She smells April and May, as Shakespeare has it, I myself can only smell danger. Yesterday D. showed her a photograph in a magazine. "Like Minty, isn't she?" he said. "Just such heavenly long legs." "Very nice," she said, as if she were talking to a child.

'We see a great deal of Charles. This leave was bound to be a strain for him. So lonely, poor man. "We must have some music one of these evenings," he said to her the other day, but I doubt if we ever shall and if they do I'll be bound Dermot will be up looking at Tom's television within two shakes of a lamb's tail. *What* a time-waster *that is*! Of course, there are some interesting programmes if one discriminates.

'To go back to Kate . . .'

She went back to Kate for a few more pages. Then, as usual, she bade her friend burn the letter (as if any of the people mentioned in it might travel down to the Cornish Bird Sanctuary and go through Gertrude's desk out of curiosity), signed it 'Yours affy, Ethel,' and sealed it.

On her way downstairs, she tapped on Tom's door to ask if he could sell her a stamp. Neither he nor Dermot had one. They were sitting there, quite mesmerised by the screen. '*Swan Lake* on ice,' Dermot explained briefly, settling back in his chair.

'I haven't skated for years,' Ethel said. 'Not since Cock Marsh used to freeze at Bourne End.' Humming to the music, she stretched out her arm and shut the door very quietly and then sat down on the edge of Tom's bed, beating time with her letter, happily enduring the smoky atmosphere.

Mrs Meacock's spirits—whose fluctuations Ethel had noted—rose as the warm weather continued. Her appetite improved: it was a great disability to her when she had none. The menus she suggested became more and more American to match the sunshine; salads, to Dermot's dismay, were full of pineapple, meat sweetly glazed; corn fritters abounding. 'I could never take to the curries in India,' she told Kate. 'One is supposed to feel cooler after eating them, but I couldn't fancy them in the first place. Cold weather food I call them, and so they are.'

As she gently stirred a pale green soup, she wore the smug expression of an expert being watched by the unskilled; self-conscious in the most pleasurable way of being so. She would not have minded Kate leaning there against the table indefinitely.

'We must have Vichyssoise one day when Mr Thornton is here,' Kate said. 'I know he dotes on it.'

'A peculiar word to choose—"dote",' Mrs Meacock thought. 'My American family always said it was strange that it took an English woman to make a really good Vichyssoise.' She pronounced it differently to correct Kate's attempt. 'That's that,' she said. She put the soup into the refrigerator and turned her attention to some sweet corn.

'Cooks never mind praising themselves,' Kate thought. 'No false, or any other kind of modesty inhibits them. The most they concede is to say "Although I say it myself", at the end.' 'How is your book coming along?' she asked.

At once Mrs Meacock looked uncertain and she frowned as she broke an egg into the basin of sweet corn, and seemed vague, as if she were not sure of what she was doing. Literature, it was obvious, bred less confidence than cooking. Among its ingredients one could be lost. 'I've too much material to manipulate,' she said. 'That's my trouble, I think.'

'Surely it is better than the other way round?'

'That I've never suffered from, so I couldn't say. Prolixity is *my* problem. Having too much, you see.' She took up the pepper mill and turned it once or twice over the mixing bowl. 'I've been a great reader all my life. One tends to have a wide range at one's finger-tips.' Kate was glad to see confidence returning. 'With an anthology,' Mrs Meacock went on, 'there are several modes of approach. I've plumped now for the chronological—in order of time, that is. It has its own problems, but once they're sorted out it should be plain sailing.'

'I do so hope it will be,' said Kate.

Her words were no comfort to Mrs Meacock, whose deep fear was out of reach of such conventional encouragement. 'What is the use of it? Where is the point?' were the words she fought against in secret. They welled up now at the back of her mind, as clearly as if they were in print. They had a physically chilling effect on her. If they were unanswerable, she would never escape again. The anthology was her loophole, her way out to places where nothing but foreign words fell peacefully about her and people's clothes were as strange as the vegetation. The sky here—at the height of summer, at noonday—was the palest blue; the colours of the Thames Valley were insipid to her—gentle, like a Beatrix Potter illustration. Tame, she thought, yearning for a blinding white temple against a gentian sky. To stay in this house for years and years, seeing nothing but the faint greens and greys of their famous view, would kill her spirit, and she would not allow its possibility. 'If one begins listening to the devil,' she decided, 'nothing will ever be done. It just leads to silliness, from one absurd question to another, until one ends up wondering what was the use of writing *War and Peace*, for instance.' She regarded that as the ultimate achievement, as a sacred novel almost, about which, like the Bible, there are not two opinions. One subscribed to it, or kept quiet. She herself subscribed to it, although she had not read it. She seemed to know all about it without doing so.

Both women gazed at the basin as she stirred. The mixture was now of a dropping consistency and she put the spoon down. 'Well, that's that,' she said.

Kate took up her sewing basket and went out-of-doors. There Dermot stood talking to the old gardener, who meanwhile kept his face averted—it was a sardonic face with skin drawn tightly over the bones, like the smiling death-mask from Mycenae. Kate sat down on a seat and opened the basket. The piece of white linen she took out to mend dazzled her eyes and she shifted round to hold it in her shadow. Threading a needle, she listened with amusement to Dermot, who was trying to persuade the gardener to spray one of the mildewed trees. The old man made only a few scornful interjections; for nature took its toll, he implied, and was bound to do so. After a while, his toad-like hand crept into his jacket and he brought out a large silver watch on his palm and stared hard at it, trying to make Dermot understand that it was twelve o'clock and time for his dinner. Pretending to mistake a pause for the end of the conversation, he made off across the garden.

Kate lifted her head and smiled. 'You can't win,' she said.

'It's too hot to argue.'

Dermot stood looking at the view. Beyond the sloping garden, the wide valley lay in a haze; the nearer orchard was full of glinting tin to keep the birds away. On the other side of the railway track, the rose-red building estate was like a blurred flower-bed when he half shut his eyes. The Castle was lost. He stood behind Kate, with his hand on her shoulder.

'It is like a summer in a book,' Kate said.

'Or those I remember as a child, in Ireland.'

'It may be only *one* summer we remember—an exceptionally good one that stands for all the others. It's the same scene, the same place in my memory and I the same height always. I could stand right under the branches of the buddleia and watch the butterflies getting drunk.' She lifted her eyes from her work. 'The hot weather, and I was bored because the grown-ups rested in the heat. I knocked the croquet balls about on the lawn all by myself, or spent my time eating Victoria plums and having diarrhoea.'

He drew her shoulders back against him and slid his hands inside her thin shirt. At once, she dropped her sewing into her lap and closed her eyes, hit unexpectedly by vertigo, by desire. For a second, pressing her head back hard against him, she wildly thought that she must have him take her, there, at that moment—with the house in view, Ethel at an upstairs window perhaps, Mrs Meacock tripping out for some mint, or the gardener returning for something he had forgotten; but the extreme sensation, when it had seemed to swing her dizzily into the air, dropped her again. She felt weak, as hollow as an empty shell, and he counted her heartbeat settling slowly to its usual pace. He took his hands out of her shirt and stroked her hair.

'You take me too much by surprise,' she said.

'I'm glad.' He sat down beside her and she began to sew again.

'It has been a day for surprises,' said Kate.

Plans and surprises had been sprung upon her while she was having her breakfast. Edwina had finally goaded her son into making an arrangement to preclude once and for all her schemes for bettering her acquaintances—such as Lord Auden—with, via Dermot, a helping of Kate's capital. A chance meeting with an old friend had led him to the very thing he thought he wanted, and he could begin working in London as soon as ever he wished. That Kate's money was involved in this project, too, there was no need to mention for a week or two. After the trial period they would discuss a partnership.

He had read his friend's letter to Kate as she sat in bed drinking coffee. He himself paced restlessly about the room, telling her of his plans, the money-spinning travel agency in Bond Street, the bright prospects, since every single person in the British Isles would soon be taking his holidays abroad. 'You can't go wrong,' he said—a phrase he more often used in connection with horse-racing and which, to her, had a ring of doom about it. 'I said nothing while I was uncertain, though my mother drove me into dropping hints.'

Kate wondered what Edwina would have to say, and could hardly believe that she was not behind the scheme. 'What exactly will you have to do?' she had asked him.

'Well, I'll be in charge of what they call public relations.'

'It is better than intimate,' she said, and this had put another idea into his head and he had taken away her breakfast tray and got back into bed with her.

'You're quite sure you think it's a splendid notion?' he now asked her as she sat beside him on the seat, sewing busily to take her mind off sexual desire.

'I can't expect to have you cooped up here all day for ever and ever, much as I should like to,' she said, as tactfully as, on this both hot and lusty morning, she could. 'You will have to get a handsome new London suit. I wonder what time you will come back in the evenings—which commuter's train? Shall you wear your bowler hat? I shall come down to meet you at the station and feel a real suburban wife again.' Her last word was ill-chosen and she would have liked to have snapped it off as she snapped off a piece of cotton between her teeth. 'I must have some new plans for myself,' she said, looking about the garden. 'I am in the mood for improvements. Shall I throw out a bow window or build a patio?'

'If you want improvements, you should begin with that old car.'

The intensity of his scorn for their car was something she could not understand. 'It gets us from A to B, as they say,' she replied.

He often wondered who 'they' were. She was always quoting them. People like himself, he guessed. Getting from A to B was to him the least important thing and he was irritated that she spoke so dispassionately about the car, did not feel her self-esteem lowered by it and could forego, from indifference, the heady pleasures of both driving fast and being envied. He often read out to her advertisements for the kinds of cars in which he had more faith, or questioned her safety in driving the one she had; and Tom supported him if he was there. It was the time of year for selling, they explained, and wondered why she any longer needed what they called—in tones meant to be disdainful—a family car. 'After all, Lou's hardly ever here,' Dermot now said, his thoughts having arrived at that point along a well-worn trail. But he intended to be patient with his nagging campaign and cut short today's part of it, priding himself on his tactics.

'What's for lunch?' he asked her, like a child.

8

'You ought to be paid overtime for it,' Dermot said.

Tom, having changed into his best suit, was returning to the factory for a cocktail party. Dermot, also in his best suit and carrying a briefcase, had come from the station with Kate. She, in her cool gingham dress and sandals, looked the one to be envied.

'That stifling train, all the sweaty city men,' Dermot said, as he and Kate got out of the car and Tom got into his. He had, coming home from work, a delightful sensation that he was acting in a play and that the rôle was well within his range.

'What's in that briefcase?' Tom asked him.

'An evening newspaper for your mother,' Dermot replied, and opened the bag to show him. 'Knocking badly, today,' he added, nodding at the bonnet of the car.

'I'm not surprised,' Tom said. 'I must rush off now and hand the drinks round to the customers.'

'He should attend to those things in business hours,' Dermot shouted, as Tom started the engine. 'Tell him from me. Otherwise, he should pay you time and a half. Of course, I speak as a worker,' he said to Kate, as they walked towards the house. 'Today now, I've fixed up a trip to Bangkok for a lady of eighty-three. She took to me at once, you know. "You'd charm the birds off the tree," she said to me, "and now you're charming me all the way to Siam." I must go and tell Mrs Meacock all about it. Don't you think vicarious is better than nothing?'

'No, I don't,' Kate said. 'I think it's worse.'

Tom, already late, was held up by a herd of cows. They filled the lane, jostling one another, stumbling, breaking into a panicky jog-trot, swishing their tails. A boy shouted oaths at them and whacked their dirty rumps with a stick, as Tom tried to edge his way forward, fretfully impatient. The road steamed with cow-pats and flies swarmed in from every direction.

At a standstill, Tom looked at his watch. 'It's good of you to come at all,' he could hear his grandfather saying, in reply to his apology. 'These gentlemen will feel themselves honoured.' Any subsequent drop in orders would be the result of Tom's discourtesy. 'You're not among the Chelsea set *here*,' was the latest refrain. Sir Alfred had glimpsed him on one of his bowing-out evenings with Ignazia, who was dressed for the occasion as a Paris taxi-driver.

At last, the lowing, shying creatures turned into a field gate, foolishly made bottle-necks, backed and sorted themselves out. Tom, making up for lost time, and taking a corner too fast, saw Araminta walking along the lane towards him. The sun was shining through the branches overhead and patterned her white dress with the shadows of leaves. She walked sedately, carrying a letter to the post. Because he was always looking for her and seldom seeing her, she now seemed a miraculous apparition and his mouth dried with the fear that he would mismanage the encounter.

He stopped the car and leaned out. 'It's all cow muck farther on,' he warned her. 'You'll spoil your white shoes.'

'You look very smart,' she said, peering inside the car to inspect him.

'I have to go to a party in the office block. Customers who have been going over the factory with their wives. You'd think a woman could find something better to do with her time. You'd be amazed if you could see them, they have everything—fancy spectacles, ear-rings, pearls, flowers in their button-holes, veils on their hats. Why don't you come with me?'

'It doesn't sound very nice.'

'Then you could post your letter in the town.'

'If you posted it for me, I needn't go.'

'I always forget letters.'

'And your grandfather might not like it.'

'My grandfather would be delighted.' Tom got out of the car and went round to hold the other door open coaxingly. He dared not hope that she would come, and while she was hesitating, he felt reckless with excitement. It was possible that his grandfather would never forgive him, not only for being late, but for being late in such startling company—this beautiful, half-bare creature in her scrap of a dress. The Chelsea set indeed. Dismissal in the morning, recriminations, will-altering—he could imagine it— and under the circumstances he could not reasonably expect Ignazia to further his interests with the wine-shipper.

Araminta smiled and came round the front of the car. 'If you don't mind stopping at the house for a moment while I fetch my handbag,' she said, settling herself beside him and slamming the door.

Waiting for her, with the engine running as a reminder to her wherever she was, whatever she was doing inside, he was in a turmoil of elation and despair. How, he wondered, could his grandfather understand that the God-given opportunity must be seized, remembering, as he obviously must, only the senti-mentalities of love and not its hazards?

Presently, smelling freshly powdered, she returned.

'I had to leave a note for Daddy, poor darling,' she explained.

'Why "poor"?'

'*You* wouldn't care to be old, would you? And lonely? And knowing that everything has already happened and hasn't been any great shakes either?'

This remote likelihood was *too* remote for him to heed on such an evening.

'I love to drive fast,' she said approvingly, as he shot past a lorry, swerved out of the way of oncoming traffic, cut in before a bus. They were nearing the factory and terror was in his bowels.

Beyond the big gates, the yard was empty save for a row of cars outside the office block. Exposed, as he felt himself, to the windows in the tower above, Tom hurried Araminta through the doors and up the stairs. As they reached the top, they could hear the high-pitched, cocktail-party noise, and it suddenly roared louder when Miss Parfitt, Sir Alfred's secretary, came through to the outer office, carrying an empty tray. 'You *are* expected,' she hissed at Tom, pretending unsuccessfully not to have noticed Araminta as she hurried past.

Sir Alfred was listening to a chattering little woman, who clutched a glass to her bosom, shrouding it in both hands, as if it were precious. He held no glass himself, as he preferred to drinking the power of seeing other people drink too much. His hands were clasped behind his back, and his head was inclined to the woman's rose-laden hat. He turned his eyes as Tom came in and, without altering his grave, attentive expression, flicked his fingers impatiently behind his back, motioning his grandson towards him.

'I'm sorry I'm late, sir,' Tom said, interrupting the conversation, receiving a look from above the roses full of admonition and contempt.

Araminta, without saying a word, had interrupted most of the conversation in the room. Standing very straight beside Tom, she glanced coolly about her, as if she were an invisible onlooker.

The woman with the roses fell silent and sipped her drink, waiting to be introduced.

'You remember Minty, Grandfather,' Tom said, in a voice without confidence or hope.

'The Thornton girl?' Sir Alfred looked ready to be unimpressed.

Araminta, lifting her eyes towards him, smiled. She stepped forward and placing her hands on either side of his face, went up on tiptoe and kissed him. Tom was astonished to see his grandfather blushing.

'I've known you since you were so high,' the old man said. She whispered something in his ear and he took a handkerchief from his breast pocket and, when he had wiped his mouth, put it into his trousers' pocket. 'Let me get you something to drink,' he said, leading her by the elbow away from Tom. 'Tell me, what's that silly name your parents gave you?'

'Araminta. I think my mother got it from a novel she was reading when she was expecting.'

'I've never read a novel with anyone in it called Araminta.'

'Neither have I. And wouldn't, either.'

'That wretched boy to bring you so late. I'll be bound all the smoked salmon has gone.'

'But it was I who made him late, begging him to bring me and then keeping him waiting. I knew you would forgive me—unless you had completely changed since last I saw you. I won't forget hitting you on the nose with a tennis ball when I was a little girl. You bled all over your white flannels, but you begged for me not to be scolded.'

'It was only an accident. I marvel at your remembering. Now, drink that up and have another. You've a lot to catch up. And then come and talk to some of my guests.'

'But where's your own drink?' she protested.

He quickly took a full glass from the tray and steered her gently towards one of his most influential customers, a bison-like man, husband of the woman with the rose hat. He used both hands in shaking hers, chaffed Sir Alfred, wagged his finger roguishly and directed gallantry upon Araminta with the application of a fireman playing water over an unquenchable blaze. His wife, dully watching through her veil, tried for a while to whip up some animation with Tom, but the boy was unresponsive and soon both of them fell silent. They drank and brooded, observing the ever-growing group of men round Araminta and Sir Alfred and, like most of the other wives, this one tried to price the girl's frock, decided on fifteen shillings, and went on to wonder what, if anything, she was wearing underneath. 'We were just leaving when you arrived,' she told Tom. 'I must try to catch my husband's eye. We've a long drive before us.'

'I never know what to look at when I'm listening to this sort of music,' Dermot whispered to Ethel under cover of a loud passage from the horns. He had been gazing self-consciously in one direction after another and had found himself staring with an absurd fixity at Charles's old suède shoes.

Charles himself had solved the problem—if one had existed for him—by closing his eyes, and Dermot tried this for a while, but it seemed to leave him all alone with the music. 'Surely it's awfully loud,' he thought. He recalled Tom's so often having been asked to turn down the volume when he was playing his own records—the ones Kate did not care for—and this was far more deafening. He could have wept with boredom and the buffeting his ears were getting. Trying not to fidget, he began to count some sweet peas in a bowl on the window-sill, desperately separating one from another, forgetting where he had started, beginning again, almost cross-eyed with the effort. Failing, he found it difficult to relax.

He had been surprised at Kate's listening expression, one he had never seen before, and which embarrassed him. Her brows had been lifted as if in tragic enquiry—how much more suffering must she contemplate?—and her eyes were full of sadness. She looked twenty years older and he had decided that the music did not suit her. He watched her breast rising very slowly and slowly sinking. For long periods she seemed not to breathe at all. When the telephone rang in the hall, she had gone out quickly and quietly to answer it, and Dermot wished that he had been nearer to the door to have forestalled her.

Ethel seemed happy. She sat beside him, her head cocked and the smile his whispered remark had caused still on her lips. Charles had slumped deep in his arm-chair with his legs stretched out. He might have been asleep, but Dermot knew that he was not. His hands were clasped on his stomach and sometimes one thumb tapped gently against the other to the rhythm of the music.

'He fairly laps it up,' Dermot thought, '—and he makes himself at home while he's doing so.' Sitting bolt upright, feeling uneasy, he—Dermot—might have been the guest. His eyes strayed back to the sweet peas; he turned them resolutely away, lest he should go mad, and folded his arms across his chest and looked out of the window. Without knowing, he sighed and Ethel, with her mariner's eye, glanced at him.

If there were a screen to look at it would be better, he decided. If one could actually see the orchestra doing it one's mind might be taken off the music itself. He tried to picture them—black and white sweating men, bows slashing the air, all at one angle, heads nodding, cheeks puffing out. Cymbals clashed and he started violently. They were working themselves into a frenzy. Surely—he dared hope—they could not sustain such a fury of sound much longer? The climax was such a wonderful relief and in happy gratitude he was just about to jump up and fill glasses when a single flute meandered into a solo passage; dying away, but not quite; returning with more assurance and inviting—Dermot was in no doubt—the whole orchestra to keep it company, which, one instrument after another, it did.

The end came quite unexpectedly. The music simply broke off. But crafty Charles was ready for it, Dermot observed. He had opened his eyes for the last bars, shrugged himself up in his chair and leaned forward, looking as pleased as Punch.

'It was Tom,' Kate said, returning. 'He won't be back. He is taking Minty to the cinema.'

.　　　.　　　.　　　.　　　.

When the party was over, Araminta had wandered round the room finishing up the canapés—every broken, faded bit that was left over. Tom considered this sign of hunger a good omen and turned his back and took a swift look inside his wallet; but it was to the cinema she wished to go, she said.

Sir Alfred, departing, patted her cheek. She did not kiss him again, was busily licking sardine oil off her fingers. He was surprised that habits he would ordinarily deplore did not, in her, displease him. He could not have blamed her, if they did. She had simply—Tom, too, and most young people—not been well brought up. That she was capable of learning he was positive. She was both sharp and charming in her urchin way and would do

161

Tom good, he thought; would shake him up with her energy and ambitions. She spat an olive stone out of the open window and went foraging among the empty glasses for more to eat. 'You will think I have worms,' she said cheerfully.

As he was driven homewards, Sir Alfred felt both hopeful for his grandson and delighted with himself for keeping up with the times. To be constantly censorious with the young showed lack of vision, he decided. Women had changed almost unbelievably in his lifetime; girls nowadays seemed a different species, quite differently created from those he had known as a young man; they were a new race of beings, so agile, fluid, forthright. On their toes, he thought. To him suddenly, all of England's girlhood looked like Araminta. He had only her in mind.

Perhaps poor Ethel and her friends, he thought, with all their long-ago suffragette nonsense had achieved something after all—though it had not benefited themselves. Freedom to behave in her own style was what Araminta had from them. She made the most of it. 'How does she keep warm,' he wondered.

'Are you warm enough?' Tom asked her as they entered the cinema.

She nodded, holding her nose at the smell of disinfectant.

They pushed open the swing doors and were just in time to see the Queen chatting to Lord Rosebery in the paddock at Ascot.

'Would you like to have my jacket over your shoulders?' Tom whispered, as they sat down. 'Your arms are quite cold,' he added, having nervously touched one of them with his finger-tips.

'Shush!' said someone from behind.

The Queen was joined now by several other smiling Royal ladies whose pale draperies fluttered in the breeze.

'No, thank you,' Araminta said loudly. 'I truly am perfectly warm.'

'A cigarette?'

'I will when the big film begins.'

'May I trouble you to remove your hat?' a woman, leaning forward, hissed in her ear.

Araminta turned her head. 'I don't happen to be wearing a hat,' she said. 'Aren't people extraordinary?' she asked Tom. 'Everybody in London has her hair done high like this. You would hardly think it could be mistaken for a hat. I *should* like to smoke please, after all.'

He struck a match and, cupping his hand round it, watched her cheeks hollowing as she drew on the cigarette. 'Thank you, darling,' she lightly said, and leaned back in her seat. It was the first time she had called him by this endearment, which she had in constant use for other people. 'The Monster From The Mangroves,' she read aloud from the screen. 'How perfectly splendid—it's an "X". I've longed so passionately to see it.'

'I do wish you would settle down,' a voice said from behind.

Araminta blew out smoke. 'What exactly *are* mangroves?' she asked Tom. 'Are they a sort of gorilla?'

Dawn was breaking over black swamps; from the knotted roots of trees snakes began to uncoil themselves, vultures circled high up in the air. 'What a sinister place,' said Araminta, in her clear voice. Out of the slime a crocodile poked his evil jaws, emerged slowly and lumbered towards the camera. 'Oh, just like *Peter Pan*,' said Minty. 'Do you remember, we were taken to see it together when we were small.'

Tom was conscious of tongues clicking behind them. Seats banged as people vacated them and, with exasperated murmurs and over-elaborate apologies and explanations to those that they disturbed, groped for quieter surroundings.

Araminta was laughing at the crocodile, who reminded her now of a clockwork toy she had once had. As she laughed, she put her thin hands to her cheeks, sitting straight-backed and intent, as if she had forgotten him. Leaning back so that he could look at her profile unnoticed, he could only marvel at his feelings towards her, so novel an experience they were to him—his strange lack of antagonism, of the contentions he had engaged in with Ignazia and all the other girls next to whom he had sat in cinemas, plotting the moves to come. He did not want to score over Minty or to have anything from her that she did not want to give. He knew that he would never fight duels with her, but only on her behalf if the need arose, as he wished it *would* arise.

Without turning her head, she tapped his knee lightly. 'Watch the screen,' she said.

He attempted to do so, and was repelled by what he saw. The monster, long-rumoured to lie under the mangroves, had begun to stir; there were earthquakes and eruptions and strange vapours, glimpses of a pallid, slithering, tentacled creature, which could heave itself up to a great height or lose all shape and sprawl over whole villages, asphyxiating men and cattle and poisoning the vegetation, giving off lethal emanations. The crocodile—an early victim—now lay dying from the villainous fumes, its jaws opening and shutting like a pair of scissors. Tentacles rose from the mangroves; a pale substance, in which floated two obscene eyes, emerged, poured through the tree roots, quivering like an enormous jelly-fish.

'Actually, it's made from tripe,' said Araminta, 'or so I read.' Tom felt queasy. He could not believe that it was tripe. It was an evil and nauseous efflux and he shrank from it. Pouring down mountain sides, and then reassembling itself, it lay in wait for innocent lovers out walking in twilight who, warned too late by the dread miasma, were trapped and sickeningly engulfed. Araminta sat entranced, her hands now clasped loosely in her lap, Tom, unable to share her simple pleasure, closed his eyes and when, once again, Minty touched his knee, he started violently.

'Do watch the screen,' she whispered. 'Surely you're not bored?'

'No, wind up,' he said.

'I promise you it will come out all right in the end.' She took his hand and held it comfortably in hers. 'Is that better?' she asked him, smiling encouragingly as if to a nervous child and then returning her attention to the screen.

Their clasped hands rested on her thigh and by flattening his palm hard against hers, lacing their fingers together, pressing the pulse beat at her wrist, he sent her messages she seemed not to receive. When he moved his hand towards the inside of her thigh she almost automatically replaced it.

The monster was a silent creature and while he was on the move there was no music to accompany him. He was now slithering down mossy steps to the burial vaults from whose dead he drew his loathsome sustenance.

'It's strange that I don't really mind him at all. He's only a cosy old thing who can't help himself,' Araminta said. She thought it a great pity when one of the corpses climbed out of a coffin and drove stakes through his eyes, the only vulnerable part of him, as she explained to Tom, who, from both fear and love, had fallen behind with the story.

They stood up for 'God Save the Queen'. 'How wonderfully thrilling,' she said, while this was going on. Tom, from soldiering habits, stood stiffly to attention and moved only his eyes in her direction. 'Could we have some fish and chips?' she asked.

.   .   .   .   .   .

'I am so sorry if the music bored you,' Kate said.

'Sorry *for* me, that it should have done, you mean,' Dermot suggested.

He let her think that his mood was due to boredom, but it was a worse and more long-standing malaise that he was suffering from —the dissatisfactions with himself—that dogged him. He sometimes wondered at what point it was that he had lost his self-esteem. To be conscious of loss proved that he must once have had it, but he could not remember the time. He told himself that his uneasiness was out of all proportion to his faults of character, for he could not think of anything really evil he had done. Other people committed worse sins and seemed to live at peace with themselves.

At times, his instinct was to say his prayers, although he no longer believed in God. He had not so much rejected his religion as lapsed from it, and he was still superstitious over this matter as he was with others, and tempting Providence seemed to him the most alarming folly.

How would Kate react, he wondered, if he were suddenly to kneel down beside their bed in prayer? He had never been able to pray unless kneeling and with his eyes shut tight. Even so, it was hard work. She would be embarrassed, he decided. She would pretend she had not seen.

Kate was in bed already, lying on her side with her back to him. She wore no nightgown in summer. Her arms were crossed on her breasts and one hand with its red-painted nails hung over her freckled shoulder-blade, her bracelet dangling its medallion down her back. She was thinking about Lou, as she usually did before she fell asleep. At least her thoughts were less anxious during the summer term, when she did not have so much to be pitying about, not having to picture to herself the cold dormitory, the boring winter's walk on Sundays—she thought of Lou most of all on Sundays—the darkness after tea, the chilblains and the frozen playing fields.

If she were still in an apologetic turn of mind about the musical evening, Dermot felt that it might be a sensible time to bring up the matter of the travel agency and its lack of capital. He did so and she listened to his voice but not to what it was saying, for she was fretting now about the school food and its deficiencies. Lying with her back to him she looked out at the starry sky. She could smell the night-scented stocks in the garden. The air was warm and the bedclothes light upon her and she turned her thoughts from Lou and began to count her blessings instead. She was always mystified that this should comfort her so little, for she was sure she had so many more than other people.

In the middle of his exposition, Dermot suddenly asked, 'Have you gone to sleep?'

'No. Why?'

'You were so quiet.'

'I was looking at the stars. I wish I knew all their names.'

'I hoped you were listening to me.'

'I was doing that, too.'

'Well, then, what is your opinion?'

'Can't we leave it for another time? Business matters always bother me. Let's ask Charles about it some time.'

'Why Charles?' he coldly asked.

'He knows about these boring things,' she said, exercising tact too late.

He lay in a huffy silence.

When she reached out and touched him lightly with the back of her hand, he ignored her.

'Tom is most terribly late home,' she said presently.

'He so often is,' Dermot replied, shifting a little away from her. 'He's not a child.'

The difference tonight was that he was out with Araminta, he supposed.

'They say, you know, that one cannot hear bats crying after one is middle-aged. The sound is too high for one's narrowing range,' she said chattily. 'I find it reassuring that I still can.'

He sighed.

'I was thinking about the old car,' she went on. 'I am sure you are really quite right about it. If we have a new one, what kind do you think we should have?'

He noted her concession, but as she had made it he decided to return to it at another time of his own choosing. 'You could ask Charles,' he said. 'I think I must go to sleep now, if you don't mind, or I shall never want to get up in the morning.'

Kate thought, 'He has worked himself bitter, as home-made wine will do.' She lay awake for a long time, listening for Tom. The stars, strung out above the trees, began to lose their brilliance and the sky paled, too. At last she fell asleep.

Tom walked up the drive, treading silently on the grass verge, let himself in quietly and crept upstairs. The house was night-quiet. They were all as fast asleep as innkeepers of an afternoon. They dreamt their innocent, middle-aged dreams and rested their ageing bones.

9

'THE thing is,' Tom began at breakfast the next morning, 'how am I to get to work?'

It was a family breakfast again, now that Dermot went to London and Kate drove him to the station. She, finding it difficult to get back into an early-rising habit, dressed hurriedly and always hoped to make the journey without meeting anyone. She dreaded winter, with its cold and dark mornings, but at the back of her mind, believed the situation would have changed by then.

'What is wrong with your car?' she asked Tom. She had just come downstairs and was going through the letters, hoping for one from Lou.

'I've explained it all to Dermot. To cut a long story short I had trouble with it last night and had to walk home.'

'What about Araminta?' she asked, looking up from the letters.

'Araminta had to walk, too.'

'You were terribly late. What on earth is Charles going to say about it? Don't tell us you ran out of petrol, please. Where did it happen?'

'Along Long Wood Lane. I did not run out of petrol. You must be thinking of your own heyday. Dermot and I both think the timing has gone. But what Charles has to say about it is my very least concern.'

'Do you mean the car just stopped as you were driving along?'

'I was able to pull in off the road.'

'Oh.' She looked at him and then lowered her eyes and began to slit open an envelope. 'Well, I shall have to drive you to the factory and you must send someone to tow your car in later. You really look as if you haven't been to bed at all.'

'If I may say so, you look fairly shagged yourself.'

'I'm sure that word meant something improper when I was young.'

'Times change.' He looked at her with what he thought of as a level gaze. 'But if it was so improper, should you have known it?'

Ethel, who thought breakfast-time a test of character, was interested by what this one was revealing.

Love was turning Tom hostile to every other person but one. They all affronted him by cluttering up the earth, by impinging on his thoughts. He tried to drive them away from his secret by rudeness and he reminded Ethel of an old goose she had once had, who protected her nest with such hissings, such clumsy ferocity that she claimed the attention of even the unconcerned.

'Gracious living,' thought Kate, who pined for her leisurely bedroom breakfast and looked with distaste at the cluttered table —at the scattered newspaper, crumpled envelopes, fallen-over packets of cereal, and empty grapefruit peels into one of which Dermot was pressing out a cigarette end.

'We had better be off,' he said. He shot his wrist out of his cuff and glared at his watch in what Ethel always thought of as a subaltern's gesture. She could imagine him tapping his leg with a cane as he did so. He stirred memories of what Lou had called 'the old-fashioned war'.

Kate drank her coffee, reading at the same time a boring and reproachful letter from an old school friend in Rhodesia. It was a report of material progress, of large cars driving great distances to parties, of new verandas being built on, of shopping expeditions to Salisbury. She had 'hectic week-ends' and 'coped with chores' and still had time to write these long letters to Kate who rarely answered them. This one Kate screwed up and aimed at the wastepaper-basket.

Dermot had gone to fetch the car. There was a sudden confusion, of things remembered at the last minute, reminders shouted, doors either slammed or left wide open. When they had gone, Ethel sat down again and swallowed some rose-hip tablets and read her horoscope. For those born under Capricorn it was to be a splendid day—for travelling, for entertaining, for speculation. 'Such nonsense,' she thought, smiling peacefully.

When Kate returned with the shopping, she stood for a moment in the hall and listened to the house humming round her, above her. The refrigerator broke into a whirring noise, overhead the vacuum cleaner bumped over an uneven floor, a kettle began to whistle furiously in the kitchen and Mrs Meacock ran downstairs muttering to it that she was coming.

The telephone rang and Kate put down her shopping basket and lifted the receiver. 'Charles here,' said his voice. 'Are you busy? Could you waste some of the day with me?' She was blushing and turned her back as Ethel came into the hall. 'Will you come for a walk?' he asked. 'I want to ask your advice about something.'

'I haven't even made the beds.'

'I will come in about half an hour.'

She hesitated still and he said, 'Tell them you won't be back for luncheon.'

That last word sounded so formal and elderly. Neither Dermot nor Tom would ever have dreamed of using it. Keeping up with the times, they whittled away at their vocabulary while Charles was padding his out.

'I shan't be in for lunch,' she told Ethel, who was setting out to take her dog for its usual morning, sniffing, leg-lifting amble; and before Ethel could reply, Kate hastened to the kitchen and said the same thing to Mrs Meacock. They had planned one of their men-absent meals of hash or rissoles and Mrs Meacock was already concentrating on the evening, making a salmon mousse for the first course.

When Charles arrived, Kate was ready and hoping that they might set off before Ethel came back. Disturbed by a dream, still carrying it about with her, she felt uneasy and had earlier blushed at the sound of his voice for that reason. She kept her eyes lowered as they walked along the road and would not ask any questions about his plans for the day. She guessed that in the canvas bag he carried over his shoulder was a picnic lunch for both of them and she thought how ridiculous Tom and Dermot would think it for a man to pack up sandwiches and carry them about in a satchel. What they could not have carried in a pocket they would have left at home, but the occasion could hardly have arisen, as they never went for walks.

Ethel was ahead of them, on her return journey, standing patiently waiting by a telegraph post. As soon as the dog had all four feet on the ground, she hauled him on towards them, waving gladly as if she had not seen either of them for a very long time and was tremendously surprised to do so now. Charles greeted her, Kate stood by smiling vaguely, then Ethel went on her way, back home to write a letter to Gertrude.

Father Blizzard went by on his bicycle, but he seemed to be wrapped up in his thoughts and did not notice them. They climbed over a stile and crossed a field. Little patches of silver river glittered through the woods far away in the valley. It was beginning to be hot.

'Poor Dermot stuffed up in London,' Kate said.

Dismissing Dermot's plight, Charles said, 'I wanted to ask you about Minty. It was some fine old hour that she came in this morning. I simply didn't know what to say about it, so I said nothing. It was the sort of thing I should have left for her mother to deal with.'

'Tom had trouble with the car.'

'Well, quite.'

'He really and truly did. He left it down the lane here and I had to take him to the factory this morning.'

'The point is, she has to go to London and she looks tired out. If it happens again something will have to be said, but I can't think what.'

'Let's see if they've towed it away yet. He said he pulled it in off the road somewhere along here.' They had come to Long Wood Lane, into the shade of the beech-trees.

'You look tired yourself, Kate,' he said, but in the same tetchy tone of voice. In her ludicrous dream, he had been more tender; he had looked at her with sympathy, then sternly with love, he had put his hands on her breast—Charles, the familiar stranger, he had been until then, no subject for conjecture or speculation, best friend's husband, no man more forbidden. Waking, she felt shocked and flurried and pressed her hands to her breast as if his were still lying there. Waking more fully, she was ashamed. The dream, although no effort of will, had subtly changed him in her mind. She had wanted him changed back again, but she had been content to lie awake for a long time afterwards, tracing the dream back to its beginning. It had hung about her since. Meeting him was a matter of embarrassment.

He had stopped suddenly and was staring up through the woods where a grassy, rutted track made its way between the trees. 'I'm glad he managed to pull it off the road,' he said.

At the end of the track, by a farm gate, Tom's car had sunk into a ditch, its wheels had scuffed up the black leaf-mould and entangled themselves in long grasses and loops of briar.

'Darling, there's surely no need to look so grim,' said Kate. 'We were young once, too.'

'Darling' had long been a permissible friend's-husband form of address, but now, after all these years, it seemed suddenly changed and she wished she had not used it.

'Don't let's interfere, or even say we've seen the car,' she went on. 'It would be silly to antagonise them.'

'I'll swear she wasn't in by four o'clock this morning,' Charles said. He gave one last worried look at the car as they walked on. 'She was as waspish as could be this morning. I shouldn't have believed it possible. All I could think was that Dorothea would have known what to do about it.'

And Tom, too, had been cross, Kate said.

Women can conceive children at any hour of the day, she would have told him if she could have found the courage. Four o'clock in the morning *or* afternoon. It was plainly this that worried him, not Minty's tired face or cross-patch mood. She felt herself in a delicate position and was afraid to brazen things out on her son's behalf, or to be so confident as to tempt providence and have her words thrown in her teeth later.

'Well, why should *they* be bad-tempered? It ought to be our prerogative in the circumstances.'

'Tom is in love with her. To him, we are all monstrous encumbrances, senile creatures littering up his path.'

'Minty is overtired,' he insisted, dwelling on the safer issue. 'That's perfectly plain.'

'I do hope she's in love, too,' Kate thought. She could not bear it for her son if the girl were not. She said, 'It's strange how sympathetic one can be to young lovers in literature and yet react so irritably to them in real life. Wouldn't one fend off Romeo from one's own daughter? I wouldn't have him within a mile of Lou if I had any say in it, the unstable youth. What behaviour! And that naughty, forward girl.'

'I blame the mother,' Charles said.

They turned off the lane into the sunshine and could see the river again and the white wings of sailing boats tipped rakishly as they moved slowly between the water meadows. There was a haze over the valley and a weekday peace. Overlooking this view, Charles and Kate sat down at the edge of a wood and spread out their picnic. Cold cutlets were unwrapped from the stiff, monogrammed napkins Dorothea had once kept for her most impressive dinner parties, hard-boiled eggs from a crumpled paper bag. As one of the wine glasses had broken they both drank from the other. 'It is simply bliss,' Kate said, handing it back to Charles. She meant the quiet, the sun, being with him, the gentle and reassuring landscape, as well as the wine. Dorothea's death had scarcely altered the friend's-husband constraint, and her dream had thrown up other barriers, but she intended to take each moment for what it was, as she took each mouthful of wine without anticipating the next.

'Food tastes better out of doors,' Charles said. He threw away a cutlet bone and wiped his hands on the grass. 'Or in bed. Alan used to smuggle parcels of fish and chips to the dormitory at school . . . I can smell them now and feel that warm, greasy news-paper . . . soggy bits of hake inside curly batter and long, bendy chips. We used to lie there stuffing ourselves, using our navels for salt-cellars. It was worth a whacking . . . or seemed so then. Bliss. as you say.'

A new thing learnt about Alan, thought Kate, who at one time had hungered for any extra detail, however trivial the recollection, to add to the knowledge of him that she was left with. Charles, who had known him since their schooldays, had been her chief source of comfort, and he had gone on filling in the picture for her and searching his memory until the same need rising for himself made him forget.

She refilled the glass and handed it to him, holding it carefully turned one way. He put his hands over hers and twisted the glass round so that he drank from the place her lips had touched. Unable to forget her dream—which hung about her like a stubborn cold—she hoped that he would not sense through her tingling fingers the embarrassment she was feeling, and when he had finished drink-ing, she drew her hands quickly from his and raked her mind desperately for something casual to say. Only the weather came to her rescue, as it always does to English people. Even hotter than yesterday, she observed. Not a sign of a break . . . she gave a know-ing glance at the sky . . . and it had been the best summer for two hundred years, she had read. 'Shelley had no idea what an English summer could be,' she said. 'I imagine him walking by the river down there, in indifferent weather, with just a picture of summer in his mind, one got from foreign parts. Born too soon, he and the rest.'

Charles lay back with his hands clasped under his head, and she knew that he was looking at her, although her own eyes were fixed with great attention upon the view. She affected an alertness, as if she expected curious happenings to be enacted at any moment in the tranquil fields below. She sat upright, plucking the grass busily, but the sun and the wine had made her limbs, and even her eyelids, heavy.

'Talk to me about Dermot,' Charles said. Her surprise at his words made her turn her head quickly to look at him.

He propped himself on an elbow and began to play a teasing game with a beetle, barring its way with a twig until he realised how demented it was. 'Are you happy?' he asked.

'Very happy,' she replied.

'Good. That's what I want you to be.' He threw the twig away and let the beetle run into the grass.

Kate was conscious of all bliss dissolving, of a stain upon the day, now that—reminded of Dermot—she realised how little she wanted to tell him about her outing. The thought troubled her enough to make her forget the objective pose, the alert expression. Charles noted the change in her and, sitting up and beginning to pack up the picnic things, he asked, 'You are telling me the truth, Kate?'

She nodded.

When everything was cleared away and the egg-shells stamped into the ground, he stood up and helped her to her feet. Taking his hand, she thought, 'It is bound to be like the dream and I could not bear the embarrassment.'

He let go of her hand and lightly brushed some dead leaves from her skirt. Leading the way back through the wood, he held aside briars for her and trod down nettles. Following him, she felt an enraged shame, as if she had put her thought into words and been rejected.

. . . . .

Tom, whose car had been fetched for him, drove home slowly through the factory traffic. Bicycles seemed to weave about him like a web and only when he came to the foot of the hill did he drive faster and disentangle himself. All day long he had felt enmeshed, trapped in unreality. He had believed that being in love enhances one's surroundings, but had discovered that, on the contrary, everything looked more flat and drab, not worthy of his exaltation or ready to match his mood. Echoing voices had been both meaningless and hurtful. When he had dropped a spanner on his foot—and he had been clumsy all the morning—he had felt the most alarming pain, as if his nerves were lying on the surface of his skin and his bones were as soft as a baby's. 'That's the third time you've dropped something,' one of his workmates said. 'He's in love,' said another. 'Haven't you noticed how he keeps looking at the clock?' This was so, and he could not help himself. The day he regarded as a hiatus, as all time spent out of Araminta's company must now be, he thought.

He waited at the top of the station slope, got out of the car, and stood, with his elbows on the parapet of the bridge, looking Londonwards. The train was due and wives were driving up to meet their husbands; cars were parked all the way down the slope. On the up platform a porter stood waiting beside a hamper of live pigeons. The signal came down with a sudden rush like a guillotine, making Tom start violently. He wiped his forehead with his handkerchief and felt himself beset, suddenly and at this last minute, with desperate necessities—to slake his thirst, pass water, wash his sweating hands. He could only comb his hair, which the wind immediately ruffled.

The train's smoke appeared above the trees, the porter moved forward and the wives started up their cars. Dermot was one of the first to jump on to the platform. He turned and gave his hand first, with great care and gallantry, to an elderly neighbour and then, with less care but obviously more pleasure, to Araminta. They were laughing as they went towards the ticket barrier; they had an air of commuters' camaraderie. Guiding her through the crowd at the gate, he put his hand on the top of her arm and kept it there as they crossed the station yard.

Tom went quickly down the slope to meet them. He tried to have two expressions on his face at the same time—of welcome for Araminta and of stern admonition for Dermot, who simply thought—as Araminta did—that he looked harassed.

'Have you got your car back?' Dermot asked him.

Tom ignored this question and put out his hand for a large wicker basket that Araminta was carrying.

'She won't let anyone take that from her,' Dermot added. His proprietary manner angered Tom, who had forgotten about his being on the train and had looked forward to a different kind of meeting, alone with Minty.

'Where did you leave your car?' he asked her.

She changed her basket from one arm to the other. 'I didn't bring it. Usually, Dermot gives me a lift in his beautiful new car—'

'She finishes her breakfast on the way to the station,' Dermot said. 'Bread and runny honey this morning and it trickled all over the seat. May I suggest that we get ourselves a drink?'

'We haven't time,' Tom said. 'Minty and I are going out.'

She looked surprised, but followed him to his car. Dermot left his in the station yard and crossed the road to the Railway Tavern. He turned and waved to them before he went in through the door marked Saloon.

'Horrible, fusty place,' said Tom.

'I am quite thirsty though,' Araminta said.

'We can do better than that.'

She threw her basket on to the back seat and settled herself in the car. Her dark silk dress was high-necked and the tight skirt was slit at the sides. It was her pale, Oriental make-up that Charles—thinking it caused by fatigue—had worried about that morning. Business men, hurrying by, all glanced into the car with great interest, Tom noticed.

'What have you been doing all day?' he asked.

'I had my photograph taken wearing a nightgown in a high wind. It wasn't really windy, of course, but the photographer's assistant held up the back of the nightgown on some pieces of cotton, to make it look as if it were billowing out. There was a mass of artificial ivy and a broken old statue. All very blurred and romantic. Quite hideous. The sort of trousseau nightgown that bridegrooms are supposed to find so kindling. I wouldn't be seen dead in it. Or perhaps "dead" is just what it's right for. It would look touching in a coffin. Where are we going for our drink?'

'Down to the river.'

'Oh, good.'

She was so brisk, that last night's kisses might never have happened. It was a worrying prospect if, at each meeting, he must begin at the beginning again.

'I thought we might have dinner there,' he suggested.

'By the weir? How lovely. Please may I have smoked salmon? I will gladly pay the difference.'

He smiled and took her hands.

'I so enjoyed last night,' she said, and might have been saying thank you for a dinner party, he thought.

.   .   .   .   .

It was almost dark when they left the hotel after dinner and they walked for a little way along the towing-path, hand in hand. 'Wonderful smoked salmon,' Araminta said.

Her tight dress was creased across the tops of her thighs from having been sat in. It was obviously a dress—a cheongsam, she called it—for wearing while standing bolt upright. Stepping out of the car, she had lengthened one of the slits by several inches.

When they came to the Lock they turned back. The air was heavy with scent from the Lock garden. Pale tobacco flowers showed up in the darkness beyond the white painted chains. A thick mist was rising off the river banks and they moved through it, feeling like ghosts.

'Two beautiful evenings, one after the other,' Tom said, in a voice no one had ever heard before.

'Such fun,' Araminta said.

They drove homewards, climbing from the valley, between high hedges. When they came to the crest, they left the car and walked through the trees, out on to the little plateau where Kate and Charles had earlier eaten their picnic. The mist had blotted out the river, but above it lights were shining on the slopes.

'I mustn't be late home,' said Araminta. 'Isn't the grass damp?'

she asked, when he asked her to sit down. She did so with some difficulty, easing her skirt above her knees.

'I love this dress,' he said. It was becoming less and less of a dress and tore again when he tried to embrace her.

'It's a cheongsam.'

'Yes, you told me,' he murmured hurriedly.

'I shall have to cobble it up in the morning,' she said, hearing more stitches giving way.

'Don't think about the morning.' He clasped his hands round her throat and said, 'Dermot did this once and I was furiously angry. And I always shall be where you're concerned. How many other people have made love to you?'

'Absolutely none.'

'I'm so glad. I wish you were only mine now and for ever. I wish you would marry me.' He looked at her with the anxiety of love and she looped her thin arms round his neck and leaned against him.

'I don't know you well enough,' she said.

'But you've known me all your life.'

'I didn't like you though.'

'I'm terribly sorry about your dress,' he said, for it had torn again.

'It doesn't matter as long as only the seams are going. I can soon mend it.'

'It was a pity you made it quite so tight.'

It was a strange conversation, he thought—he whispering and her voice sounding so clear and loud in the still air.

She sat bolt upright with her back to him. 'You could undo it,' she suggested in the same distinct voice. She was so expert, so decisive that he could not help asking her again about other love-making. In France? in London? he wondered.

'Absolutely not,' she said, wriggling her shoulders free of the loosened silk. 'Wouldn't it be dreadful if anyone were to come? Could one be sent to prison? I remember having picnics here when we were children. Someone else has been. There are egg-shells.'

He took off his jacket and spread it out upon the ground. 'I simply mustn't be late home,' she said again. Now she was busy with her hair, repinning loose ends as if it were morning and she were just going off to London. Its neat, Oriental arrangement made her look both prim and exotic.

'Do you love me more now than you did when you say you didn't love me at all?' he asked.

'I think I do. I'm sure I do. Well, it could hardly be possible not to.'

'I'm so glad.' He felt quite ill with gratitude and amazement. 'You're sure you aren't cold, my darling girl?'

She gave her hair a last pat and then lifted her arms wide like a triumphant orator acknowledging applause, and Tom leant into her embrace and lowered her on to the warmness of his coat—a hallowed garment to him from then on. 'It's quite a mild night really,' she said.

[10]

'IT's the loveliest of all in Horse Show Week,' Lou told Charles. 'When it's floodlit at night and looks as if it is floating in the sky.'

Obediently, he trained the telescope on to the Castle, but the sun went in suddenly and the ramparts became a blurred shadow which only Lou, who knew it so well, could distinguish. Still holding the telescope to her eye, while trees and far-off cottages swam in and out of sight, he said, 'I saw you coming out of the church this afternoon.'

She had dropped in to pray for her mother and had found Father Blizzard there, talking to some workmen about the boiler. ('I am relegated to the more domestic chores,' he had explained when the men had gone. 'I am cumbered about with much serving.')

'I went there to pray for Mother,' Lou decided to tell Charles.

'For any special reasons?' He turned his head slightly, looking down at her.

'No.'

He also made a quick decision. 'Because of the other night?' he asked. Lou, taken by surprise, burst into tears. Hoping very much that no one would come in, he put his arm round her and she pressed her wet face against his rough jacket. When the weeping eased off, she groped for the handkerchief in his breast-pocket, keeping her face hidden against him. 'May I?' she asked. He gave her the handkerchief and she wiped her eyes. 'Do you mind if I blow my nose?'

'Help yourself.'

'I'm very sorry I cried.'

'I'm sorry there was any cause.' He turned back to the telescope again. He found her distressingly pathetic, with her rough, clumsy ways, her bewildered air. 'It sounds patronising,' he continued, 'but I shouldn't be unduly put out. They probably have compensations you can't begin to imagine.'

'Oh, sex, you mean?' she said aloofly.

'And other things.'

'My father would never have sworn at her—especially not in front of us. I'm quite sure he wouldn't have done it at all.' Charles said nothing. 'Do *you* think he would have done?'

'No. But people are different.'

'And it probably went on after they had gone to bed. Her eyes were very red in the morning. So that's why I go into church now every day. I've often said prayers for her, but so far I've had no luck.'

'I should keep pegging away.'

She looked at him sharply, thinking he was making fun of her, but he was squinting through the telescope and his lips were set firmly together.

'I think things are going from bad to worse,' she said. 'Every time I come home it seems that they are. "Bloody smug." Fancy saying that to her. My father would turn in his grave. And then, when she went out of the room, he said it again, and Mrs Meacock must have heard him.' She was beginning to dramatise the incident and he wondered if the crying had done her good or harm. There was a risk that the air had been cleared too much.

'Best to forget it now,' he said. 'He was really cross with himself.'

'For being drunk, you mean?'

He lowered his voice nervously and said, 'For upsetting the wine-glass, and being caught out in a harmless lie.'

Lou had a sudden, indignant feeling—which she at once realised was unreasonable—that he ought not to have entered into this discussion of them in their own house, in their absence. Despite their lowered voices, she felt uneasy, and kept glancing at the door.

'Dermot's the one you ought to pray for,' Charles said.

'He's supposed to be a Roman Catholic. He should be praying

for himself. Oh, there's his car. You can hear it coming from a mile away. Do I look as if I have been crying?'

'I think anyone might guess. I should keep your head turned, or look through the telescope.'

'You would think the new car would have made him happy. He talks to Tom of nothing else—on and on, as if he's simply compelled to. It seems almost indecent, the way he drags it into every conversation. It's a fixation,' she said, in a condescending tone of voice. 'It's like exposing himself.'

'Have you got us all weighed up?' Charles asked.

'I do know one thing—he'll be embarrassed at meeting you again after the other evening.'

'I thought so, too. That's why I called in. I was afraid that if I left it too long he might imagine I was embarrassed too.'

'And are you?'

'A little, but I mean to get the better of it. Can you tell me what that little white speck is high up on the left of the Castle?'

'It's the War Memorial at Runnymede. Charles, do you think that Minty is in love with Tom? He is with her, you know.'

'Ah, that's a whole new field. We'll have to go into that another day.'

She sighed with pleasure at the thought, much steadied and cheered by their conversation.

'That was that nice little curate you were coming out of the church with?' he asked. 'Father Something doesn't he call himself?'

'Blizzard. I pray for him, too. The whole village is up in arms about him.'

'Really? Nothing has come to my ears.'

'They say he goes too far; too High, they mean.'

Charles imagined him soaring away—a black, flapping kite. From below came the menacing shouts of villagers. 'Are there enraged discussions among the commuters? Denunciations in The Bird in Hand?' he asked. He wondered who could really be concerned about the poor fellow—one or two Low-

Church old ladies, perhaps. And dear Lou, for different reasons.

'The Vicar keeps saying, "If you want a thing done properly, you must do it yourself." And he gives him all the most boring jobs. Father Blizzard says that he is really no better than a Verger. Any minute now, he expects the Vicar to ask him to mow the grass in the churchyard, or ring the bell for early service. Anything to keep him away from the altar.'

'Was he saying all this to you in the church this afternoon?' Charles asked in some surprise.

'No, outside.'

'And why is he so dangerous that he mustn't go near the altar?'

'He elevates the Host,' Lou said as the door opened and Dermot came in.

'Good evening, Charles,' said Dermot, with a great deal of Irish geniality in his voice.

Louisa moved at once to the telescope to have her back to him.

'Where's Kate?' asked Dermot.

'She's gone down to the farm for some eggs,' Lou said. 'Mrs Meacock used eight in that apricot mousse. Mother says she will have to be curbed.'

'I ought to go,' Charles said vaguely, glancing at his watch but not noting the time. 'I just dropped in . . . I thought you got back earlier.'

'There's no hurry surely? I took your daughter for a little drink. She had some liver sausage in her basket and some cheese that stank to heaven.'

'She is always eating liver sausage,' said Charles, and he sighed, as if he were speaking of a serious malady.

'She was even nibbling at it in the pub,' said Dermot. 'A very hungry girl.' He turned towards the table where Mrs Meacock had put the tray of drinks. 'What will you imbibe?' he asked, smiling to himself as he took up the decanter. He picked these phrases with care and uttered them precisely and maliciously, watching keenly for a sign from Charles—for the slightest flicker of distaste; but Charles stayed bland and vague. As the glass of sherry was handed over, their eyes met for the first time that evening, and it was Charles who looked away first.

'The most astonishing good health to you,' Dermot said, lifting up his own drink. 'I'm sorry, Lou. Do you want anything?'

'I don't drink.' She brought the hazy Surrey hills into range. Even she was growing bored with the beloved view, but she dared not turn round.

A door banged. There were voices in the kitchen, and then Kate came bustling in. Ever since a few evenings before, when Dermot returning drunk and late for dinner had spoken harshly to her, she had moved in a bright little whirlwind of her own making, with not a minute to spare for anyone. She was always on the wing, setting out on one errand after another, and no one could hope to detain her or say a word that would be listened to. Their words were what she dreaded— their thoughts she knew—and, trapped at mealtimes, she warded them off with a torrent of her own. The flow was more easily come by when she had had several drinks. In attaining this end, Dermot, full of uneasy contrition, was ready to encourage her.

'I had to go down to the farm,' she explained in her new, rather breathless voice. She must have hurried off when she was half-way through a drink, thought Charles, seeing Dermot take a glass from the tray and hand it to her, saying, 'Finish that and make a fresh start.' His tone of voice was indulgent but unloving. 'When will they ever thaw?' Lou wondered. Bored with the view, she had turned the telescope on to a large toad which came out each evening to crouch on the cool lawn, which she had watered earlier in the day. She thought that she would never be able to forget the breakfast that followed what had probably been for her mother a sleepless night. She and Dermot had not by then arrived at their present state of nervous brightness and they had hurried through their meal in silence, with newspapers held high in trembling hands to screen themselves, their facial muscles rigid. How could they ever begin to speak to one another again? Lou had wondered. By the time Dermot returned that evening, Kate had assumed her new manner, had adjusted her mask. He had quickly imitated her, had gone off at once to mend the garage door, which had been broken for three months. Since then, only the trap of mealtimes had threatened them. The dining-room table—like an altar to the god of family dissensions—was the place where they were most exposed, where they handed food to one another and kept their glance averted, where enquiries had to be made and silences cut short. Kate's eyes had found a middle-distance at which she could look without really seeing anyone or anything. Her bustling about the village provided her with enough trivial gossip to fill the gaps in the conversation. Lou did not feel herself called upon to help. Ethel had too little inventiveness.

This evening she—Ethel—had waited until after Dermot's home-coming before she left her letter-writing. ('Quite worn out with pouring oil on troubled waters,' she described herself to Gertrude.) She came into the drawing-room wearing her calm, oil-pouring smile, but her eyes, not having discovered the useful middle-distance, darted about like trapped animals. 'Why, Charles, I had no idea you were here.' A further embarrassment, she thought—another witness reappearing. 'What a lovely day again!'

'It seems to be clouding over, though,' said Kate.

'But still dry. Every morning one thinks that it must break.'

'We need the rain,' Charles said. 'The roses are covered with green-fly.'

'I've never known a summer with so much blight,' Ethel said enthusiastically. 'It's just the same in Cornwall, so my friend wrote in her last letter. You remember Gertrude, of course?'

Charles said that he did not and realised at once that it would have been simpler if he had said he did.

'Surely! You must remember her. One of my closest friends. We were old lags together at one time. "Now you two old lags," Alan used to say to us. That was because we were both in prison together, and loved chatting about it. How he teased us! Oh, she and I often came here together. You must have met her. She went grey very early—a well-built woman with a deep voice. As a matter of fact, she was a wonderful singer when she was younger. I'm sure you met her on several occasions when we were visiting Kate.'

Charles thought, 'I wonder how people would describe *me* in such a few short phrases—"Always dressed so untidily: couldn't pronounce his r's"—Thus, perhaps, if Ethel were talking of me. With other people, I should obviously fare worse.' 'I expect so,' he said to her. 'I just can't . . .'

'Drove a Morris Oxford car for years and years. Alan used to tease her about that. . . .'

'I should probably know her if I . . .'

'Not unlike Dame Ethel Smyth—her features.' Charles could not for the moment bring Dame Ethel Smyth's features to mind, either. 'I know Dorothea would remember at once,' Ethel said with great certainty and then, thinking 'What a disastrous thing to say', blushed and fell suddenly silent.

'That was one of Dorothea's many gifts—remembering everybody she had ever met,' Charles said. 'And everything about them, too. I relied too much on her promptings and now I'm at sea without them.'

'You're very quiet, Lou,' said Dermot. 'What have we flying over the Castle this evening—The Union Jack or the Royal Standard?'

'You know perfectly well the Queen's at Balmoral,' Lou said. 'Not that I could see anyway. Actually, I'm watching a toad.'

'It's been a very bad summer for toads,' said Ethel.

'There have been a lot about, you mean?' asked Dermot.

'No, the poor things suffer so much in a drought. They need moisture on their skins, I believe.'

'One is always drawn back to the view,' Charles said. He went over to the window and stood beside her. 'Especially in the evening when it is changing all the time. Can you see the cloud shadows across the hillside, Lou?'

'How long before it is all built over, I wonder?' said Kate.

Ethel's horrified protestations gave Charles cover enough to murmur to Lou, 'It's all right to turn round now.'

'Are you sure?'

'Perfectly.' Over his shoulder he said to the others, 'Perhaps one day Lou will stand at this window and say to her children, "I remember this when it was all fields." And they will hardly listen, they will be so bored. Especially as they will have heard it so many times before.'

While they talked, Kate was glad to relax and save her resources until dinner-time. Dermot had refilled her glass and she began to feel more confident, but when Tom came in she felt constrained again. For Tom had put into words the thoughts the others had kept veiled. Bluntly, the very next day, when her wound was raw, he had asked her, 'Are you all right?' as if the idea had suddenly occurred to him that, surprisingly, she might not be. 'You're not still upset about Dermot's being elephants last night?' This way of putting it had made Dermot's behaviour seem merely hapless, his drunkenness an endearing weakness. 'You're behaving like children, both of you, going on being so huffy. You used to be cross if Lou and I were sulky. "Wasting your days in rancour," you always said. All right, I'll say no more.' She had not spoken, but her disapproval and annoyance were plain to see. 'Wasting your days in rancour,' he had repeated to himself as he turned to go. 'It's funny how phrases get buried in your mind for years and years and then surface all of a sudden.'

He had not brought up the subject again. He let matters slide, though making no pretences, as the others did, that nothing had happened. Something was still happening and he was deeply conscious of it. He did not alter his own behaviour in any way and his exuberance this evening was the natural expression of how he was feeling—a rare thing lately amongst them.

'Are your glasses charged?' he asked as soon as he had slammed the door. 'The unimaginable has happened to me, so you can all be upstanding.'

Lou, who, in spite of Charles's assurance, had not yet risked showing her face, forgot herself and spun round quickly. She was sure that Araminta must have said that she would marry Tom and, before he had uttered another word, she was half-way up the aisle behind her, wearing mauve.

'My grandfather has suddenly warmed to me,' said Tom. 'My humble days at the bench are over. I am to be transferred to the Sales Department—missing one or two rungs of the ladder on the way there, I am pleased to note. There I shall be, with a nice clean job, no more cheek from those foul-mouthed girls in the canteen, lunch with the executives, who have known me since I was a little lad, they say. Mr Tom, they will call me.'

'I'm so pleased for you,' said Kate.

'What about money?' Dermot asked.

'That, too.' Tom gave him what he thought of as a sage look and turned to pour himself out a drink.

'I'm so pleased, darling,' Kate said again. 'You have been very patient. I'm glad he's shown such confidence in you.'

'Confidence! We had a ceremonial lunch at The Chequers. The last time I was taken there I was taken there for ticking-off purposes. But today every delight was displayed before my startled eyes—a bottle of Krug, salmon in aspic . . . I've got to learn how to entertain customers, you see . . . beautiful bonuses, undreamt-of freedom on the Board . . . his own blissful retirement . . and after that the Chair itself. Nothing impossible. Am I talking too much?'

'It is only what you were intended for,' said Kate. 'There is no one else to follow on, but I could never make you understand how much that meant to him. He had to put you through the test.'

'Well, all the time, I thought I was hanging on by my finger-nails. Never doing a right thing. Clumsy young oaf, spoon-fed dilettante, welfare-state delinquent. I've been the lot. Teddy-boy, because my trousers were cut too narrow: crummy Chelsea set, because my hair was too long, and a bald-headed G.I. when I had it cut short. Now everything is changed. All of a sudden he seems to think the sun shines out of . . . that I can't do anything wrong. I do believe I could even grow a beard and get away with it.

'Oh, don't, dear boy,' said Ethel quickly.

Charles said, 'I'm very pleased for you, Tom. Congratulations. And now I must get back to my dear daughter.'

As he left the room with Dermot, Tom's eyes followed him, as he himself would like to have done. His excitement ebbed and he sat down on the edge of the sofa and sipped his drink, staring in front of him. Thinking that everyone had gone from the room to see Charles off and that he could safely brood and look pessimistic, he sat hunched up and frowning, exhausted with his worry about Araminta. He was reminded of the exasperation he had suffered as a child when a balloon had floated away from his grasp. He would reach it, but as soon as his fingers touched it, it would bob on ahead of him, until, broken with fury, he had screamed and thrown a stone at it. If he couldn't have it, he would rather it were destroyed. 'But I don't want Minty hurt,' he thought. 'Not even if I can't have her.' The impotent rage was the same as his childhood's, but now he knew about love and that it was necessary to have patience. 'But I get nowhere with her,' he told himself and thought how strange this conclusion was, considering how far on several occasions he had been allowed to go. Even so, at the next meeting, as at every meeting, he would be faced with her chilling friendliness, as if nothing at all had happened; whereas he felt himself to be so changed that he half-expected to be berated for the very expression on his face, poor exposed creature that he was.

He sighed and then started when Lou, who was still standing by the window, suddenly spoke to him. He reassembled his look of optimism and emptied his glass. 'What did you say?' he asked.

'I said, "It's strange how Minty stays thin."'

'Why?'

'If she eats all that liver sausage.'

'I don't know what you're talking about.'

'Dermot was saying she had bought some liver sausage and Charles says she's always eating it.'

'Oh? When was this?'

'Just now. Dermot brought her home from the station.'

'Then I hope he drove carefully. He's a maniac in that car.'

Further discussions with his grandfather had delayed him and when he had arrived at the station the train and most of the cars had gone and the platform was deserted. She never waited.

'I can't understand how any girl loses weight when she's in love —all those meals they get taken out to. I remember how Ignazia got thin, in spite of all the smoked salmon you bought her. I saw her in the town the other day. I think she looks top-heavy now that she's lost her stomach, don't you?'

'Hm,' said Tom. He picked up a magazine and turned its pages.

'Whereas Minty is thin all the way down. I rather admire her figure.'

Tom appeared to find the magazine absorbing, although it had such a domestic and feminine approach. He was reading the letters and advice column and found it enlightening, although what 'Worried', who was asked to send a stamped and addressed envelope for her reply, was worried about interested him very much.

'Do you?' Lou asked.

'Do I what?'

'Admire Minty's figure.'

'A bit too much,' Tom said. He read another letter and then looked up at Lou and said, 'I should advise you to fall in love with a fat man when the time comes. It's too agonising when you love a thin person. You're so terrified all the time that they'll snap in half.'

'Plump people can worry you, too,' thought Lou.

Tom, although still staring at the magazine, was now recalling how he had seen Araminta in London a day or two ago. She had taken a job modelling clothes in a large store. During luncheon and tea, she walked between the restaurant tables, entrancing the husbands of shoppers—their reward for a trying day with their wives—bestowing on them the friendly smile which Tom found so chilling and they so gracious. Tom, after a visit to his dentist in Portland Place, had gone to the restaurant for tea. Instead of at once finding a corner table from which he could have a good view of his beloved, he had found himself, greatly embarrassed, standing in a queue at the entrance, held back from the delights of the pink and crimson room and all its cosy chatter and tinkling sounds, by a tall woman who seemed to be receiving invisible communications from within. Occasionally, she would allow a couple of women through, pairing people off—'Do you mind sharing?'—and she seemed surprised when at last it was Tom's turn to be dealt with. 'How many?' she enquired. 'I am on my own.' 'Do you mind sharing?' 'Yes, I do, rather.' Coldly, she asked him to stand aside for a moment. By the time he reached his small table by the window, where he could look down through gauzy curtains at the glittering street and the tops of buses, he felt hot and indignant. Apart from being so out of place, he was suffering from an injection the dentist had given him. His top lip was swollen, seemed huge and clumsy, and when he put the teacup to his mouth, was not where he expected it to be. He spilt tea down his best tie and shirt. At that moment, he saw Araminta in lime-green linen and white gloves, stepping gracefully between the tables. She walked with quick little steps, one foot before the other, and occasionally touched the pearls on her bosom with one hand and deftly turned round on her toes to show off the back of the dress and her tanned shoulders. She came to Tom's table, paused for a moment, still wearing the same smile, and said, 'What a nice surprise to see you!' She did not look in the least surprised, and he wondered if this were part of her professionalism. His puffy lips tried to shape an explanation, a reason for his being there, but by then she had gone. He had taken out his handkerchief and, dipping a corner of it in the hot-water jug, began to sponge his shirt. Later, she had returned—after a matronly woman had gone sedately through the restaurant in dove-grey—a morale-lifter from the Outsize Department. As Minty came towards him the second time, he leaned forward to watch her. She was wearing a mustard-yellow coat and, approaching him, held it open to display the dress underneath. 'Isn't it ghastly?' she asked him through teeth still parted in the well-known smile. 'Don't I look a hundred in it?' She had swept on and, gazing after her, he had wondered how anyone of such fragility could possibly last the day. 'It is her neck which is the most touching,' he was thinking this evening, sitting on the sofa and staring at the photograph of a kedgeree in the magazine he was holding. 'Especially the back of her neck.' Staring at it, as she preceded him into pubs, he sometimes wondered if it could go on indefinitely supporting the weight of her head.

'What's the matter, Lou?' he asked her, glancing up as she went to the door. 'Your face looks a bit odd. You haven't been crying, have you?'

She shook her head and went into the hall. Hearing her running upstairs, Tom shrugged his shoulders.

. . . . .

The moment Charles had gone, Dermot and Kate had parted company. He had made his way to the garage and she had looked into the kitchen where Mrs Meacock was dishing up. She did not know how much Mrs Meacock disliked being visited at this stage. Straining vegetables, lifting joints from the hot oven, she liked to be alone and unfussed. It was not the most elegant part of cooking and she felt herself put out by having an audience, even if it was the mistress of the house. She stooped and picked up a glazed carrot which she had dropped and put it carefully and ostentatiously into the waste bin. If Kate had not been there, she would have popped it into the vegetable dish, thinking, 'What the eye doesn't see, the heart cannot grieve over.'

'It smells good,' Kate said with vague approval, leaving her at last in peace.

'She *is* at a loose end,' Mrs Meacock thought. 'It just shows money can't buy everything. At least I've got my peace of mind, which *she* hasn't. When I lay my head down on my pillow at night, I know I've got my peace of mind. And I wouldn't be without it, or beholden to anyone.' She took the crown of lamb from the oven, and when she had set it down, passed her hand over her forehead and her moist upper lip. It was hot, cooking. Her clothes were sticking to her. 'Oh, for five minutes with the paper,' she thought.

.   .   .   .   .

Ethel went up to her room to add a few more lines to her letter, as dinner for some reason seemed delayed and the party in the drawing-room had broken up. She rubbed her fingers over the smooth nutmegs she always carried in her pocket to ward off rheumatism, and considered the next sentence. She wished to drop a hint to Gertrude that a visit to Cornwall would be acceptable at this time. 'Things have gone beyond what I am able to put in a letter,' she wrote, after a little hesitation. 'Harsh words have broken more than bones in this house lately.'

.   .   .   .   .

Dermot stood in the garage looking at the new car. He would have liked to have got into it there and then and driven at great speed in no particular direction, but away from where he was. To do so would lift his spirits as nothing else seemed capable of doing, now that he was cut off from Kate; cut quite adrift by his own folly—as he could admit to himself and would have admitted to her if she had allowed him to. The trouble was not a mere lovers' tiff, or one of those rifts between married people smoothed out soon enough by an apology, a word of contrition. At first, he had told himself that it was. But now he could not. 'I hurt her self-esteem—and in front of Charles and the children,' he thought. He expected that she prided herself on never having wounded his, but all the same he knew the pain of it.

11

'My brain is dwindling from disuse,' Father Blizzard said to Louisa. 'I attempt to exercise it while I perform my menial tasks, but the signs are that atrophy has set in. Of course, it's not just for that reason that I've decided to leave, to ask to be released.'

He had come out of one of the almshouses as Lou, with Ethel's dog for an excuse—and having seen his bicycle outside—passed by for the third time. Following his movements lately, she had noticed that his sick-visiting, or visiting of any kind, was among the humblest cottages and poorest families. The Vicar himself made the other calls—upon the new people at the Manor, the rich old ladies on the Green and the commuters' wives in what Kate called the Underwriters' Georgian colony, those expensive houses set well back in gardens full of magnolias and flowering cherry-trees. The Vicar was snobbish she had decided; but she kept this to herself, lest Father Blizzard should find her snobbish for having had the thought arise. 'We are all God's children,' he might beg her to remember. None the less, it was plain to her that, however God regarded his children, the Vicar had his own ideas of the order of their importance.

'Do you want to know how to cure warts or varicose veins or something called white leg?' Father Blizzard asked her. 'Because if so, I am the one who can tell you.' He had been sitting in the stuffy almshouse parlour for more than an hour. There had been a pungent smell of ointment and the old lady had insisted on un-doing a sore leg for him to see. There was something watchful and obscene about her manner of doing this, as if she were testing him, expectant of squeamishness, or vindictively punishing him for what she had to suffer. He detested wound-showing, though the wound itself would not upset him. 'It can't do *her* any good,' he had thought, leaning forward dutifully. And when he left, he could not help wondering what other sort of young man would be obliged to spend half an afternoon listening to old wives' tales of sickness and travail.

'I had a letter from a friend of mine in France,' he told Lou as he bent down to fondle the spaniel's ears. 'He is studying with the Dominicans at a place near Paris. The countryside is lovely by all accounts, not far from the Seine and at the edge of a forest. I can imagine it, in this summer weather . . . such peace. He is to take vows.' As well as the wild, silent countryside, he could also imagine his friend sitting in a bare room, studying Greek or Theology—things of the mind—while he himself sat in an ointment-smelling parlour listening to talk of wart-charming and the histories of long-ago sicknesses. 'Not that one should be envious,' he said, determined not to be.

'I can't think what it will be like when you go away,' said Lou.

'I shan't leave many sad hearts behind me, I'm afraid.'

'Mine will be sad.'

'Well, thank you, Louisa. As long as there is one. I am lucky to have that.'

Pushing his bicycle, he walked beside her homewards. He had made up his mind to see the Vicar after tea, as soon as he returned from his hospital-visiting. All the afternoon, he would have been in and out of private wards, sitting amongst the grapes and carnations, brought tea by Sister herself. He was an interfering man rather than a helpful one, more harassed than compassionate. 'He means well', was the phrase most often used about him. To Father Blizzard he seemed like a collie dog, driving the sheep towards the Good Shepherd, fretfully rounding up stragglers and exhorting them with anxious geniality.

'When you go away, would you write me a letter to tell me where you are?' Louisa asked.

'Of course I will,' he said, and began to compose it at once: 'Dear Louisa, as I write this letter I am sitting at a window in the sun, looking out over the fields towards the edge of the forest. . . .'

Lou felt heavy with depression, the afternoon had a stale air and yet was precious in the light of those that were to come after. She would no doubt look back on this occasion as one of great fulfilment—to be walking beside him, for him to have confided in her —and she advised herself to make the most of it. It would seem wonderful when she had nothing else. Yet the present time was nothing if it could not last or come again: in fact, it scarcely existed. 'Look thy last on all things lovely'—a line she had hitherto delighted in with the delicious sadness possible only to the young, now struck her with its true brutality; it invoked desperate images —a man glancing up at the sky on his way to the gallows, or herself soon to take leave of Father Blizzard. 'On all things lovely,' she thought. 'He is hardly that. But lovable. He is one of the people *I* am able to love, and the only one who takes any interest in me.'

At the end of the drive he paused, took off his spectacles and wiped them on his handkerchief. 'The air is full of blight,' he said.

'Won't you come in to tea?'

'No, I have someone coming at five to borrow a dog collar for the Dramatic Society play.' He blinked kindly, looking so like a plucked owl without his spectacles, she thought.

'Are you very short-sighted?' she asked, for everything about him was important to her.

'I have unilateral amblyopia,' he said.

She was trying to remember these words as she walked up the drive, meaning to go straight to her dictionary when she reached the house. But she was hindered by Charles—who also took an interest in her, though she hardly realised it. He stopped and spoke to her as Kate was seeing him off, and the words were forgotten.

12

THE mornings now, on the London-bound platform, had an autumnal haze. 'A nip in the air,' neighbours said to one another, strolling up and down to keep warm, lifting the *Financial Times* in greeting. 'I think we must say good-bye to summer at last.' 'We can't grumble.' They seemed to believe that good weather was deserved and that England for once had had its just reward. In the station yard, behind the railings and the estate agents' posters, rusty golden rod and some pale Michaelmas daisies were strung with heavy dewy cobwebs in which sat leggy, striped spiders. School trunks—also signs of the season—were piled on the platform morning after morning now, and the commuters paced about between them, waiting for the signal to drop, spinning webs of small talk from their mouths, spider-like. 'Must lift the dahlias. Never had such a show. I hear the Somerses went to the Riviera and didn't have a single dry day. Same in Spain, the Willises said.'

Araminta snuggled into the honey-coloured mohair coat that Tom had given her for her birthday. Inside the warm, wide sleeves she clasped her elbows. She gazed with dreamy distaste at the shabby school trunks, recalled with morbid horror her own. Poor Lou. Any day now, she supposed. 'When does Lou go back?' she asked Dermot, for something to say.

'Tomorrow morning. Glad I'm not her.'

'And I. There *are* people who like it, though.'

'Lou's not at an age to like anything.'

'I was the same when I was sixteen.'

'Difficult to believe. Perhaps *she* will suddenly blossom, then.'

'Well, she's long-waisted. That's the main thing,' Araminta said with an aloof air. She sometimes wondered about Dermot.

She had several times met him or caught sight of him in London when she was making her way from her agent to a photographer or doing some shopping and once, when she was posing on the steps of the National Gallery, wearing a Persian lamb jacket she abhorred, she had seen him sitting on a seat, dozing, at three o'clock in the afternoon. She had suspicions that he merely pretended to go to work. He never had anything to say about it, took no papers from his briefcase to study on the train as most of the other men did.

'And poor Kate hasn't a clue,' she thought. If she had been a married woman herself, she might have felt a wifely fellow-indignation. As it was, she was simply rather amused.

'Are you busy these days?' she asked him.

'Fairly. Rich old ladies beginning to think of winter cruises, you know,' he said vaguely.

She nodded and went on staring at the school trunks. 'Well, rather Lou than me,' she said. And then the signal came down and she turned her thoughts to London and the day ahead.

.   .   .   .   .

In the afternoon, Ethel went through her wardrobe in preparation for her visit to Gertrude. This visit had been much postponed, for Gertrude had been so busy with her birds. Life at the sanctuary was what she herself called 'hectic'. There were sick gannets in every bedroom, or injured gulls or oil-fouled cormorants. She, with her bird-watching, seemed to have a fuller life than Ethel with her people-watching. And things had been extra quiet in the house lately. Kate's former briskness had slowed down and a morning had come when she had allowed her eyes to meet and be held by Dermot's. She had smiled a little awkwardly and blushed. 'He must have taken the bull by the horns last night,' Ethel wrote rather confusedly to Gertrude. She was glad that it should be all peacefulness at the end of Louisa's long holiday; for she had her own little sorrows, the poor child. Her attachment to the Curate—who was leaving the Parish (and the Protestant Church, too, if rumour was correct)—was obvious to Ethel. She had suffered from similar attachments in her own young days and was sympathetic of the desolation that ensued. She was sympathetic towards Tom, too. He had given Araminta an expensive coat for her birthday. To Ethel it had seemed an odd present—they were not even engaged: there had been no talk of it—and it was obvious, she had written to Gertrude, that Charles had thought so, too. 'Poor Tom,' she added, 'and what does *she* give *him*? Nothing, obviously. Not that I advocate immorality,' she hastened to make clear, 'but there is a cold and calculating virginity about the girl that does not augur well. Tom is like those sailors who will not learn to swim, for fear of a slow death. Drown he nevertheless will, unless she gives him a hand ere long. Or even a melting glance.' This last phrase had seemed rather novelettish, though, and not likely to go down well with Gertrude, so she had scratched out 'melting' and written 'kindly' above.

She decided to take one cool dress to Cornwall, in case there should be a St Luke's Little Summer later on. 'Otherwise I'll plump for woollies,' she said aloud. She shook a maroon-coloured cardigan and a nutmeg fell from the pocket. She replaced it and then took out her heather-mixture coat and skirt. It had been a wonderful long summer, but how pleasant it would be to wear her dear old suit again—so beautifully made such years and years ago that it would never wear out. With pride she examined the neat sprat's heads at the top of each pleat and the Cairngorm thistle pinned permanently to the lapel. At the sight of it her dog, who was lying on the bed, lifted one ear questioningly. 'Ah, you think you're going walkies, don't you?' Ethel said. 'Soon, we'll be going rides in chuff-chuffs,' she promised. 'And you're going to be a good boy with the birdies, aren't you?'

How still the house was. Outside the gardener, bow-legged as an old stable-lad, swilled down the yard. She could hear the water tossed out on to the flags, the bucket-handle clanking, then the harsh broom scraping the stone. Downstairs, Mrs Meacock whipped something in a basin with a fork. Ethel imagined her standing at the kitchen table, staring before her at far-off lands.

'She won't stay long,' she thought. She seemed to have given up work on her anthology, to have lost heart, reading newspapers instead. Ethel had often found her going through the advertisements of situations vacant. 'She may go off as a cook somewhere abroad,' Ethel thought. 'She won't stay here. That's certain sure.'

Going to the window to examine the seams of a pair of pewter-coloured stockings, she saw Kate sitting on her usual seat under the monkey-puzzle tree. She was doing some last-minute mending for Lou and when she saw Ethel at the window she held up a pair of bottle-green winter knickers in which she was threading elastic. She made a grimace and laughed. 'She looks happy enough,' Ethel thought. 'For the time being.'

.   .   .   .   .

Louisa waited in the church porch to say good-bye to Father Blizzard. Although so shortly to leave, he still had his menial duties. Not belonging anywhere at present and likely to profane the church with images or incense or prayers to saints, he was kept out of mischief as much as possible with widely scattered errands. It was as if the telephone had never been invented, he thought, as he set off on his bicycle with little notes to be delivered about the village. At this moment he was moving the sheaves of corn for the Harvest Festival from one place to another. Someone—who sounded to Lou like Miss Buckley—was directing him. He was obviously, from her tone of voice, out of favour with her, too.

The stone porch was cool, even chilly, but the sun was bright in the churchyard. Bleached, dry grass was tussocky on old graves, yellowing leaves floated down from the lime-trees. Pigeons were cooing. Lou had studied all the notices, knew the list for flowers off by heart, imagined Mrs Shotover three weeks hence, arranging the last of the Michaelmas daisies while she, Lou, was out doing some boring school shopping, hanging about bookshops, buying envelopes. She began to study an old balance sheet for the second time—'Wafers and Candles £5 11s. od.' she read. 'Communion Wine £3 15s. od.'—very little, she thought. 'Poppy Wreath

12s. 6d.' The wreath was still propped against the War Memorial; faded, rather, since last November.

Mrs Shotover was also in the church, for Louisa could now hear her voice, too—more motherly than Miss Buckley's—commiserating with Father Blizzard. 'Poor man, that's women all over for you. "Why can't they make up their minds?" That's what you're thinking, aren't you now? "First they ask for it to be put down here and then they want it shifted somewhere else." You'll be glad to get shot of us, I don't doubt.'

'It was Vicar's instructions,' said Miss Buckley. 'Farmer Foley was asked to leave them by the font in the first place.'

'You'll be smothered with chaff. Your black suit, too. Here, a minute.'

Lou imagined her brushing him down, smacking his shoulders with her great red hands. She turned back to the balance sheet and began to add up the expenditures.

'You will remember not to put any ears of wheat round the pulpit, won't you?' said Miss Buckley. 'Because of Vicar's hay fever.'

'Look at that great stripey marrow,' she heard Mrs Shotover exclaim. 'It looks for all the world like my old tabby cat.'

Lou felt nervous waiting there. Even the uneasy, bubbling sound of the pigeons made her more anxious, reminded her of her fluttering stomach. She hoped that he would come out of the church alone; but unfortunately, when at last he did so, he was followed by Mrs Shotover and then by Miss Buckley.

'Now, if we'd known you were here,' Mrs Shotover told her, 'we'd have dragooned you into moving some of the produce for us. Look at poor Mr Blizzard, he looks as if he's been under a haycock fast asleep, like Little Boy Blue.'

'We should welcome some help on Saturday,' said Miss Buckley.

'I'm afraid I shall be back at school by then.'

'Well, then, we must wait till Christmas,' Mrs Shotover said. 'If you're a good girl, I might let you help me decorate the font.'

'That's a great honour,' said Miss Buckley.

'And one that means nothing to me,' thought Lou, waiting for them to go, praying for them to go.

'Come and see the sheaves of corn,' said Father Blizzard. He stretched out an arm behind her back, urging her into the church and seeming to bar the others from it. 'Good-bye, Mr Blizzard,' both said.

Lou heard them crunching off down the gravel path. The church was even colder than the porch and smelt of damp stone.

'They will make a great parish worker of you,' Father Blizzard told her. He kept his voice at its usual pitch—though it had a sad note—but Lou, murmuring something—she knew not what—lowered hers, being in church. 'You can't see God for the jumble in the end,' he said, walking towards the vestry. She followed him slowly. He took a key from under a pew cushion and unlocked the door. He unlocked the outer door, too, and opened it to let the sunshine in. Lou looked round at all the hanging surplices and cassocks, and some ugly mortar-board-like hats the choir girls had to wear, and then she leaned back against a high desk and watched him searching through an attaché case.

'I am so glad I saw you,' he said. 'I had hoped to bring this to you this evening, but I have a duty call instead. I have to go to the Dramatic Society play—the one they borrowed the dog collar for, d'you remember?—and make an appeal for the church fabric in the interval. Some tedious, old-fashioned play . . . I've forgotten what . . . I expect the clergyman will be the usual silly-ass kind. People will give me sly glances to see how I'm taking it, so I'll have to laugh my head off.'

'I suppose everyone is being very difficult?' Lou asked timidly.

He had straightened his back and stood looking down at his dusty shoes. In one hand he held a little cardboard box. 'I think the Vicar is relieved and he'll be even more so when I've really and truly gone. Being, of course, most broad-minded about Rome—"dictates of conscience . . . each man's privilege and duty . . . but, none the less, if I may say so without appearing bigoted . . ." You can't, I think, but naturally don't say, for, although I've heard so much about the courage of my convictions, I'm a mouse in all human relationships. Then, as you can imagine, there has been trouble at home. None the better for having been anticipated . . . tears from my mother, and I can understand those only too painfully. She has always been hard-up. To get me here'—he glanced round at the hanging surplices—'meant the most dreary economies for her. I think she thought it had been worth it when I went home —she liked going out with me in these clothes.' He looked out through the open door at the fading sunlight on the headstones. 'Her tears almost finished me, you know. Made me feel monstrously heartless, a shiftless, obstinate cad.' He sighed and turned back to her. 'Look, I bought this for you.' He handed her the box and watched her bowed head, the incredulous smile wavering on her lips, as she opened it. 'A souvenir,' he added. 'Because you have been my kind confidante.'

She took out a bracelet of fine gilt mesh and looked up at him. 'It's like the one you gave to your sister,' she said.

'As nearly as I could find. I thought you liked that one at the time. After all, you chose it. You do like it, don't you?'

She clasped it round her wrist and then stared up at him. 'Oh, I do,' she cried. 'But I can't believe it. I swear I shall never take it off.' 'Except at school, I'll have to, I suppose,' she thought. She was so moved that she burst into tears and turned suddenly and buried her face in the Vicar's surplice.

'You mustn't do that,' Father Blizzard said in alarm and thrust his handkerchief into her hand.

Walking home slowly alone, she turned her wrist occasionally so that the bracelet caught the light. She was tremendously comforted to have it hanging on her wrist. She felt that it would keep her company wherever she went. She might not see him again, but their friendship had ended with such an unexpected fittingness that she was faintly conscious of a miraculous escape. Not everybody's love was so unclouded, or so rewarded. She had words to treasure, too. 'Because you have been my kind confidante.'

As she came to her own house, she felt set apart from, higher than, the muddles of her mother's love for Dermot, or the anxieties of Tom's love for Minty. 'I am the lucky one,' she thought. 'Even at this dreaded moment I can say that for myself.'

Her mother was sitting on the seat. She was just packing up her sewing things and she jumped up when she saw Lou. 'We'll have tea ready in a flash,' she called.

'She is only trying to cheer me up,' Lou thought. 'For the reason that it's my last day.'

Ethel leaned out of the window and waved. She guessed where Lou had been and remembered farewells of her own. 'Let's have some music after tea,' she called out. 'Just to please your poor old Aunt.'

Lou looked up and nodded. Then she held out her wrist and said to Kate: 'I have this bracelet.'

.   .   .   .

Late that night Kate, on her way to bed, looked into Lou's bedroom. Milky moonlight fell through the open window across the bed. Lou lay on her back with one braceleted arm outside the covers, her upturned toes, her breast, lifted the bedclothes to make a shallow trough between. She looked as touching as Juliet on her tomb. The moonlit drapery was like a drawing by Blake. 'There should be angels,' thought Kate.

13

THE felt hats and heavy overcoats looked strange on this hot day, but the winter term was beginning, whatever the weather. Lou was given a friendly greeting by the girls waiting at the platform gate. Kate was always relieved to see this. 'They do like her,' she told herself. 'She has her own place with them.'

Effusiveness was in the air. Kate herself was drawn into it by the girls she knew. She even had a slight acquaintance with some of the other mothers—there was only one uneasy-looking father—and the brightest of smiles were exchanged. Great care had most certainly been taken over the seeing-off clothes. They would not have seen their sons off in such frivolous hats. Daughters were a different matter.

All over Waterloo Station groups of schoolgirls flocked together—their cries, their movements birdlike, as was their way of keeping strictly to their own kind. Other uniforms drew only glances of scorn. Schoolboys, returning too, were less gregarious. They stood alone at the bookstalls or thoughtfully put pennies into slot-machines, unimpressed by so much feminine gaiety.

Hilariously, the mothers joked and teased, ecstatically their daughters recounted escapades and outings, parties, holidays abroad. 'Poor Lou, I did nothing for her,' Kate suddenly thought. It is a most severe pain—the realisation that one has failed one's child, done less than one might have done; but she continued to smile bravely. 'In the Christmas holidays—she shall have a wonderful dance,' she suddenly decided. 'I'll hire the ballroom at The Chequers. If only I could tell her now, to cheer her up. I'll write instead as soon as I get home. Do we know any boys, though? Tom's friends are much too old. They wouldn't come.

And I shouldn't want the responsibility of them, either, with young girls of Lou's age.'

The platform gates were opened and the gaiety seemed to increase. The extraordinary joy of parting was at hand. Music cases and raincoats were flung on seats, lacrosse sticks and violins hoisted on to the luggage racks; the train windows were full of smiling faces; messages were shouted and reminders repeated over and over. 'Give my love to Daddy.' 'Don't forget my chilblain ointment.' 'Let me know about Coco and the puppies.' 'Tell Tom to write,' Lou shouted to Kate, who smiled and nodded. He never would. He never had done and Lou, hereafter, would not think another thing about it.

A few new girls, dazed by the hilarity, were looking quite white with anxiety. They could recognise one another by their new clothes and the little mistakes they had made in the wearing of them. They watched as the last trunk, the last 'cello were put into the guard's van. The whistle was blown. As the train began to move, the messages came thick and fast; mothers standing on the platform blew kisses; arms waved out of all the windows, so that the train curving off out of the station looked as if it had put out feelers. One of the mothers ran a gloved finger under her eye as she turned away.

'It's all so English,' Kate said to her, walking back with her towards the ticket barrier. 'I don't know how we keep it up. They *do* settle very quickly, you know.'

The woman nodded, unsure of her voice. The mothers, having handed in their platform tickets—grave now, no longer gregarious —went different ways. Kate went to the hairdresser's, where Elbaire found her uncommunicative. She failed to ask after the baby or about his holiday at Ilfracombe.

'How has it kept, madam?' he enquired. He lifted a strand of hair and looked at it doubtfully. 'The sun's played havoc with my clients,' he told her.

That morning, Kate had asked Dermot, 'Do you mind having a grey-haired wife? Shall I have it dyed?' 'Of course I don't; but do if you would like to,' he had said. He had tried to speak in an indifferent voice, lest she should think the matter was important to him; but the air of unconcern was overdone. 'It is I myself who is becoming unimportant to him,' she had decided. He had also made excuses when she suggested calling at his office so that they might have lunch together. 'I shan't be there all day,' he had said, too hastily, too emphatically. 'I have to go out to Wimbledon to see a man.' She could not help wondering if he were telling her the truth. He sat out her hurt, suspicious silence, adding nothing else to what he had said and explaining nothing.

Kate, lifting her chin, looking at Elbaire in the mirror, suddenly said, 'I am quite tired of myself. You can make me as different as you please, and dye me blonde or raven-black or auburn. And you can cut fringes or tack on chignons to your heart's content. *Carte blanche* with me today, and I'll only open my eyes when you've finished.'

'Bring Madam the shade card, Amanda,' Elbaire called out, quickened suddenly by Kate's air of recklessness and afraid lest she should change her mind.

Kate looked placidly at magazines while they worked. She copied out a recipe from the *Tatler*, though doubting that she would ever persuade Mrs Meacock to attempt it. She was even beginning to wonder if Mrs Meacock would stay with her much longer. She had noted the signs of restlessness and was quite prepared for her to pack up her belongings—all the snippings and trimmings she had collected together, the hat-box full of newspaper-cuttings and the souvenirs of foreign travel—and be off. 'I can perfectly well do the cooking myself,' thought Kate. As she jotted down the recipe for a liver pâté, she could imagine herself in the kitchen making it. 'And I'm sure we're all tired of American food,' she thought. 'Beastly waffles and maple syrup and that sickly upside-down cake.' She turned over the pages, looked at a photograph of young people at a dance sitting out on a staircase, recognised a girl she had met in the train one evening—one of Tom's erstwhiles, as she thought of them—whose name she could never remember. 'Miss Prudence Paget,' she read, 'with her fiancé.' So she had soon consoled herself with someone else. A chinless young man. A sad come-down after Tom, Kate thought.

She was so absorbed in the magazines that she was startled when Elbaire, with the solemnity of a votary, held a glass at the back of her head and asked for her opinion. Her hair, which he had draped about her head like a turban—so that she could never wear her hat —was of such a dark colour that it looked tinged with purple. It contrasted very strangely with her sunburned face. He was turning the glass at different angles so that she could view the back of her head, and, though he did not look wholly triumphant, his expression was self-congratulatory. Kate was in good training for false smiles that day and she hid her dismay with the best one she could manage and, when she thanked him, gave him a bigger tip than usual as if to compensate him for the black thoughts in her mind.

Feeling utterly strange and self-conscious, she walked towards Edwina's. She was glad that the passers-by ignored her.

No one stopped in his tracks and stared with horror or astonishment. 'People in London are used to anything,' she thought, wishing it could be the same elsewhere. Edwina, however, made up for the passers-by. Opening the front door herself—being between foreign girls, as she later explained—she gave a very good pretence of trying to hide her surprise.

Going ahead of her up the stairs Kate, who had meant to be on her dignity, could not help making explanations. 'I simply felt bored with myself,' she added. 'It's ghastly, I know. You don't have to say it is not.'

'Well, I did wonder. . . .'

Kate passed the *trompe-l'œil* panel and went into the drawing-room. 'We all make mistakes . . .' Edwina was saying.

'I saw Lou off,' said Kate.

Edwina, with her eyes on Kate's hair, said: 'Isn't it too late for tea?'

'Yes, I'm sorry. They took longer at the hairdresser's than I expected.'

'I can easily make you some if you'd like it.' Edwina permitted herself to appear dazed by the change in Kate and was beginning to unnerve her with the expression of grave doubt upon her face. 'Or shall we just have a drink? I'm sure you could do with one. It's nearly half past five,' she added, letting her eyes turn very briefly towards the clock.

'Just a drink,' Kate said.

As if reluctantly, Edwina turned her attention to a decanter of sherry. 'I'm glad you managed to look in,' she said. 'At least I know now that you're all in the land of the living.'

'You know what the school holidays are like—and Dermot's so busy nowadays.'

'Dermot?' Edwina gave her an odd look as she handed her the glass of sherry. Then she glanced away and said again: 'Well, I'm glad you managed to look in for a moment.'

Kate, conscious of all the oblique glances, said, 'I'm sorry I was so much later than I said. All this business with my hair took hours. Such a mistake, too.' Sipping her sherry, she vaguely thought that if she kept on saying this herself, she might prevent Edwina from doing so. 'I made my mind up on the spur of the moment—just feeling I wanted a change.'

'I don't blame you,' Edwina said—but as if there were those who might.

'This smart dead room,' thought Kate. What trying hours she had spent in it; but, even so, perhaps not as many as duty had demanded. The little gilt clock seemed to shiver and rustle. Edwina smoothed her silk frock on her thigh, looking pensive. 'What train are you catching?' she enquired.

'I mustn't be too late. I told Dermot that if I didn't go down on his train, not to wait about for me. He will go home and I shall ring up from the station when I get there.'

'Why, has Dermot been in London too?'

Kate looked at her in surprise. 'Well, of course.'

'I didn't know,' Edwina said, shrugging her shoulders.

'He came up to work.'

Edwina shrugged again, but said nothing. Keeping her eyes lowered for once, she reached out for her drink.

'What do you mean, Edwina?'

Without looking at her, Edwina said: 'I don't see why Dermot should be allowed to make a fool of you—as he did of me. The simple fact is that, whether he came to London or not, he did not go to work. There is no work to go to. Perhaps he hardly knew how to tell you. One could hardly be surprised at that.'

At those brutal words—'make a fool of you'—Kate's heart seemed to drop a curtsy. She stared at Edwina, who would not look at her.

'I'm very sorry, Kate; but there it is. I expect he kept meaning to tell you and put it off and off, feeling too ashamed. And so it became difficult and, at last, impossible. It's the same old story and he knows it. So he just went on pretending—going to London day after day, not going to a job, but looking for one. Not very hard, either, I'll be bound.'

'Did he tell you this?'

'Not he. I found out. I was bound to. I often looked into the offices when I was passing.'

'How long has he . . .?'

'Not long. Only a fortnight ago he came to me to try to borrow some money.'

'What for?' Kate asked very faintly.

'To put into that firm. That young man, whoever he was, was short of capital. I don't know what the arrangement was when Dermot started there—what sort of assistance he promised to be— he was as tight as a clam about that—but it was obviously not what I should consider a satisfactory thing at all. You can rest assured he had no backing from me. I have no money to play around with and I had to tell him so.'

'Why didn't he ask *me*?' Kate said, but not really to Edwina, who, hearing her bewilderment, at last looked at her.

'I thought it was best to tell you. He's my dear son and I love him very much—perhaps even more than I love Gordon—but sometimes I'm ashamed; and never more than now.'

'Poor Dermot,' Kate said quietly. 'He will hate my having found out. How embarrassing it is. How absurd, too.'

'I thought it best to tell you,' Edwina said again. However, even at the risk of his bitter anger with her, she could not have kept the knowledge to herself. 'If he didn't love me,' Kate thought, 'he would never have minded telling me. Caring about what I should think of him was what made it too difficult.' The childishness of his deception was so full of pathos that she felt tears rising in her eyes. She put her trembling lips to her glass and drank a little to relax her aching throat. 'Whatever I do or say,' she told herself, 'I must not let him seem childish and pathetic to himself.'

'Perhaps he stayed a bachelor too long,' Edwina was saying, searching for explanations that could lay no blame on herself. 'Women always spoilt him. When he told me he was going to marry you, I couldn't believe that it would really happen. Perhaps it shouldn't have.'

Kate slowly shook her head, but not in reply either way to what Edwina had said. It was as if she were waving away thoughts too strange to be admitted. Edwina got up and fetched the decanter. 'Let me give you some more. It's been a great shock to you. I'm very sorry. I hope I did right.' She put her hand on Kate's shoulder, staring down at her strange, purplish-auburn hair. 'She's trying to be kind,' Kate thought. 'But how I wish I had come to know of this without her—that I needn't share it with her and suffer her curiosity.'

'He is so different from his brother,' Edwina said. She had one satisfactory son; the world could not say that she had failed altogether. 'Gordon has never given me a moment's anxiety. Even at school, they were as different as chalk from cheese, with Gordon winning all the prizes and passing all the exams. And Dermot . . . why, the only thing he ever passed in was Religious Knowledge or whatever they call it. . . .' Kate looked up in bewilderment, but

Edwina was in full swing. 'Gordon was always shut up in his room, studying; while Dermot kicked his heels and complained that he was bored. I think it would have killed his father if he had known the anxieties the boy would cause me. And when did he last go to Mass I should like to know? Oh, Patrick would have grieved. It's hardly for me as a Protestant to goad him into going—though it wouldn't be the first time. I always tried to keep my promise over that—although to me the religion seems ... well ...' She shrugged. 'All the same, nearly any kind is better than none, especially when there are inherent weaknesses. I remember once ... he was only quite a lad ... we were by way of living in Montfort Gardens at the time ... and a letter came for him while he was out. It had 'Private and Confidential' printed on the envelope. I couldn't help wondering what private and confidential matters a boy of that age could have to do with. I was so worried that I did a thing I had never done before—or since—because the boys' correspondence was sacred to me ... I wouldn't have dreamt of looking at a letter in the ordinary way, not so much as at a postmark even ... but this day while I was making myself a cup of tea to steady my nerves, I steamed the letter open. It was an account from a bookmaker for fifteen pounds. I must have gone as white as those gladioli.'

'Edwina,' Kate said, getting up from her chair. 'I think I must get home as soon as I can.' She drained her glass and put it down on a table.

'Yes, naturally, my dear. And I hope there won't be too much trouble.'

'There won't be any trouble.'

'No, of course not. That was the wrong word. ...'

'I think I understand him, but I want to talk to him and then I shall understand completely. It is just a silly muddle—not important—and can very soon be put right.' 'Holding him tightly in my arms,' she thought. 'We can solve everything that way.'

'Thank you for telling me. It can hardly have been easy.'

'It was my duty, I felt. I did it for the best.'

Kate, looking round for her gloves, glimpsed herself in a

looking-glass. 'Oh, heavens, I'd forgotten my hair. I hope he will forgive me.' She put her cheek briefly against Edwina's. 'Don't bother to come to the door. I'll let myself out.' She wanted to run. The thought of the train journey filled her with impatience. 'I must fly to him,' she thought. 'And comfort him. As soon as I am with him, everything will be put right.' For the absurd deception to continue even an hour longer was frustrating.

She hurried downstairs, relieved to be already homeward bound. Everything and everyone was forgotten but Dermot—even Lou, and the plans she had had for her—the dance she would give, the social whirl she would somehow organise.

Edwina leaned over the banisters, rather put out by this sudden flight—though in a way it was convenient, for she was dining with Lord Auden and must dress. Kate looked up from the well of the hall and lifted her hand.

'And, my dear,' Edwina called down to her, 'he does love you. You know that.'

'Yes, I know,' Kate said and she stepped out into the hazy, evening air and slammed the door behind her.

. . . . .

The train journey seemed endless. She had missed the last of the commuters' trains and this one dawdled from station to station, half empty. It was mid-evening. At home, they would have started dinner and her telephone call would have come at the wrong moment. She imagined Dermot pushing his chair back, throwing down his napkin. She was surprised, therefore, when the train eventually arrived, to see Tom coming down the platform towards her and alarmed as well at the sight—a second later—of Ethel anxiously scanning the compartments.

In spite of imminent disaster which—seeing them both there—she was certain of, she noticed that Tom looked at her in a puzzled way, as if without full recognition, checked by something he found strange. He said nothing. She put her hand to her hair and stared at him. 'How did you know that I was on this train?' she asked.

'Mother, I am sorry. There is awfully bad news.' He put his arm along her shoulder and drew her towards the ticket barrier. 'I rang up Edwina and she said you had left.'

Ethel, suddenly seeing them, came hastening up and her face, too, reflected a brief surprise in spite of having pressing disaster on her mind.

Kate staved them off. She was conscious of great calm, holding them at arm's length; perfectly steady, she assured herself, for whatever had to come. When she had got into the car, Tom stood by her for a moment with the door open, looking down at her. 'There's been an accident,' he said. ('That is how I shall have to break it to her,' he had made up his mind earlier, and since then the words had gone on and on in his head.) 'It's not the worst, but very bad. I'm afraid the car overturned.' His voice was rough, and touching to her.

'Dermot,' Kate said flatly, as if correcting his omission.

'But you mustn't think that it's without hope,' Ethel said, leaning over from the back of the car and laying her hand on Kate's shoulder. 'He's a young man still, and the young heal quickly.'

Tom got into the car and started it up.

'Is he in hospital?' Kate asked.

'Yes, at Market Swanford. I will get you there as quickly as I can.'

'But Market Swanford is miles away.'

'I know, but that is where the accident happened.'

'So many mysteries,' Kate thought. She sat with bent head, picking at the stitching of her gloves and frowning. There had been enough that she had to ask him and now there was much more. 'All that's of no consequence now,' she decided, and Ethel saw her shrug her shoulders, as if shaking something unimportant from her. 'What is wrong with him?' she asked. Her voice sounded almost surly.

'Well, they can hardly tell, dear, till he is in the theatre,' Ethel said soothingly. 'We shall know when we arrive. Charles is over there already.'

'Charles?'

'You see, Minty was with Dermot,' Tom said and, looking up at him, she saw how pale his face was, and knew that it was not only from anxiety about Dermot that he was driving fast.

'Where were they going?' She forced out the words, hating them.

'Nowhere special, I expect,' Ethel said in the sing-song, Nannyish voice she meant to be lulling. 'I expect they met at the station or came down on the train together and went for a spin to try out the car. I remember Charles saying once how Minty loved speed. He worried about her driving so fast. Perhaps she egged him on just for the fun of it and they struck the kerb for some reason—'

'Let's leave the details until we can know for sure,' Tom interrupted her. 'Guessing won't do any good.'

The length of the drive was telling on them all. Kate felt her first, miraculous calm deserting her and now she dreaded their arrival. She watched the houses flying by on the main road and marvelled that they contrived to look both strange and familiar at the same time. A dreariness of heart, a sickness, began to un-nerve her and she feared the end of their journey. As they entered what seemed to her the icy darkness of the hospital, she walked uncertainly and Tom put out his arm to steady her. 'He is certainly dead,' she told herself, following a porter down a hideous, white-tiled passage to the Sister's office. Tom and Ethel thought so, too. They were being handed on to someone who was used to breaking such news.

Yet she looked genuinely upset, Kate noted with surprise, staring at the neat, youngish woman who stood up as they entered. She swung a chair forward and put Kate into it. 'I'm afraid he's gone,' she said gently, her large white apron screening Kate from the other two. 'I'm very sorry. It was just half an hour ago. There was nothing we could do.'

.　　　.　　　.　　　.　　　.

Kate was insistent that she should drive home and that Tom

should remain with Charles. 'If only I could drive,' Ethel said, several times. 'It would have been a little thing I might have done to help,' she thought. 'I am just a useless old woman.' Kate took the journey very slowly, as if they were in a fog. She wept silently and the tears fell over her hands as they gripped the steering-wheel. When they drew up in darkness before the house, she folded her arms on the wheel and pressed her face against them. 'Worse and worse is to come,' she cried. 'I have hardly started on it. Oh, Ethel, it was anger I felt first of all. As if there were room for that.'

For the second time, Ethel tried to comfort her for her husband's death. She had gone through the whole, unrewarding business before and could visualise the different stages lying ahead. She helped Kate out of the car and drew her close to her warm, nutmeg-smelling tweeds.

'Poor Charles!' Kate wept, chafing her hands, waiting for Ethel to find her key. 'Poor Tom!' She tried to ward off her own grief by pitying those other two.

The hall light was switched on and Mrs Meacock in a blue dressing-gown came out from the kitchen. Ethel, standing behind Kate, slowly shook her head and Mrs Meacock looked at them with strange staring eyes; quite rigid, like a waxwork; but when Ethel asked for brandy she started, her eyes flickered and she almost ran towards the dining-room.

'What is all this for?' Kate asked in bewilderment, nodding at a large suitcase with an umbrella strapped to it standing in a corner of the hall.

'Well, dear, if you remember, I was going off to Gertrude's early in the morning. It can stay there for now and I'll take it back upstairs presently.' She took the glass of brandy from Mrs Meacock and in a gentle, coaxing voice, urged Kate to drink it.

.   .   .   .   .

Tom and Charles paced about the hospital waiting-room. From time to time they would sit down on one of the benches for a few seconds, but were soon driven back to their restless wandering. At intervals, one of the night staff brought in cups of tea and they occasionally whispered a remark to one another. On the notice-board was a safety first poster with a horrifying photograph of a badly burned child, and Tom tried to keep his head turned from it, feeling nausea rising each time he caught a glimpse of it.

It was a bad sign that they had asked them to stay, Charles realised. 'One is tempted to say prayers,' he thought. 'Although I don't know to whom. But something to fill in the time, something positive to do. People invent gods they can't do without.' He wondered if Tom were praying, but he knew so little about young people. They seemed to him to be untouched by religion or politics or the state of the world. In the early thirties when Charles had been a young man they had all been more seriously involved. 'We had conscience without faith,' he thought. 'And made heavy weather of it.'

'When one has waited so long,' he said to Tom, 'one is incapable of believing that it will ever end. It doesn't seem possible now that anyone will ever come and tell us anything.'

But at that moment, the door opened and the surgeon himself came in. He was a grave, worn-out-looking man, still dressed in his green theatre gown and cap. 'She is back in the ward,' he told them. 'You could see her for a moment, but she's not conscious, of course.'

'Because he thinks it is our last chance,' thought Charles, as they followed him as quietly as they could down the dim corridor. Tom, however, felt more hopeful. He was agreeably surprised that they should be invited to see her in the middle of the night.

She was lying in a little slip ward on a high bed. Blood was being dripped into one arm and a nurse stood on her other side, checking her pulse rate. The bed-clothes were lifted high over her stomach and her shoulders were bare. There was still dirt encrusted round her ears and hair line, on her grazed forehead. She looked no more than twelve years old, Charles thought, touching her hand lightly and then stepping back. Clumsy with anxiety, he trod on the nurse's foot. She ignored his apology, calmly entering something on a chart, making him feel humble and oafish and far too large for the small, crowded room. 'We are ignorant and at their mercy,' he thought.

Araminta lay in her no-man's-land and touching her hand had been a useless gesture. No message could be got through to her, he knew; he could not envelop her in his love or tell her what a strange, bewildering delight she had been to him. That perplexing and capricious creature he had been trying to become acquainted with seemed to have vanished, leaving in her place the child whom he and Dorothea had shared. He was glad that Dorothea did not have to share this night with him. She had escaped what he must suffer and this made her seem to him a dead woman at last.

Tom stood very straight, just inside the door. His face was flushed and his eyes were bright. He and Charles spoke in whispers as if Minty were simply asleep, and they were distressed lest there should be the slightest possibility of her hearing the surgeon saying in his normal voice, 'I'm afraid she is very ill indeed.'

'If only morning would come,' thought Tom. It was the muffled night that was so frightening. It seemed malevolent to him. He had heard people using such phrases as: 'He wasn't expected to last the night.' It could not happen that Minty would not last the night, because he was willing her to do so with all his strength.

'There's nothing to be gained by waiting,' the surgeon was saying. 'You can stay if you want to, of course, but she won't come round until the morning.'

'What time could we come back?' Charles asked.

'At any time you like,' the surgeon said. He nodded to them and went off down the corridor.

Tom looked back over his shoulder before they left the room, but there seemed no point in doing so. 'She had quite a good colour,' he murmured to Charles as they went stealthily back to the waiting-room. They had decided to stay.

.   .   .   .   .   .

Kate refused to go to bed—for if she slept, she would have to wake up, she said, and that she could not bear to do—to face afresh the grief she was as yet so little used to. She sat by the telephone with a coat flung over her shoulders and obediently ate and drank whatever Ethel brought to her, except for sleeping-pills. She would ring up Edwina in the morning, she decided, and so spare her the lonely night hours. Tomorrow, Gordon would hurry to her, and prove his solid worth. Meanwhile, she waited for news of Minty and fretted sickeningly for Tom.

Instead of the telephone ringing, Charles and Tom returned together. It was beginning to be light and swallows, gathering to fly away, were noisy and busy round the eaves. She ran to the window and knew at once—from the way they shut the car doors and turned and walked across the gravel—that Minty had died. She had not lasted the night after all, and Kate was afraid to meet Tom's eyes.

He was carrying some things of Dermot's—torn clothes carefully folded and a leather case. He put the case down on a table and went past Kate and up the stairs to his room, carrying the dusty clothes.

'Poor boy,' said Charles. He went over to Kate and took her in his arms. 'Who can comfort *him*?' he asked.

Mrs Meacock came down the back stairs to the kitchen and turned on the tap. They heard the water thrumming into the kettle and then china being set out on a tray. 'It is all cups of tea,' Charles said. 'Where is Ethel?'

'Upstairs, unpacking.'

Kate turned away from him and took up the leather case from the table and opened it. There was nothing inside it but an evening newspaper and her own copy of *The Spoils of Poynton* with a bus ticket between the pages to mark a place. 'He didn't get very far,' she thought. She put it down on the table and after a moment she covered her face with her hands and wept again, held tightly in Charles's arms, until she had run dry of tears.

14

IT was on a quiet, drizzly day in the next year that Kate and Charles were married. The church still bore traces of the Harvest Thanksgiving and Lou remembered with amusement the last occasion—when she had sat in the porch and listened to Miss Buckley and Mrs Shotover decorating the font. The wedding was just a family affair and Tom, having given his mother in marriage, returned to sit beside Lou. Ethel was wearing her heather-mixture coat and skirt and had a jay's feather tucked into her hat band. 'Kate was an accomplished bride,' she decided to write to Gertrude later that day, after they had seen them off on their honeymoon in Rome. 'She took everything in her stride, making her promises before the God she does not believe in, without the slightest hesitation.' Ethel mentally rearranged this sentence several times and hoped she would remember it.

'I shan't look radiant,' Kate had told Charles the evening before. 'It wouldn't be suitable with my grey hair.' But she looked very happy, Lou thought, watching her walking hand in hand with Charles under the dripping lime-trees to the lych gate. Tom held an umbrella over them as they got into the car and Lou, bright as a new leaf, stood blowing kisses after them.

As they drove away, Kate leant forward to wave and caught—before he could change it—the expression on Tom's face. 'But he is young,' she comforted herself. 'His sadness can't be for ever.'

THE END

virago

To find out more about Elizabeth Taylor
and other Virago authors,
visit our websites

www.virago.co.uk
www.viragobooks.net

for news of forthcoming titles and events,
exclusive interviews and features, competitions
and our online book-group forum.

And follow us on Twitter @ViragoBooks